The Heartbeat of Life

A Guide to Mastering Cardiopulmonary Resuscitation Techniques to Save Lives

Isabella White

Disclaimer: *The information contained in this book is based on the research, opinions, and experiences of the author. It is not intended to replace professional medical advice or treatment. The reader should regularly consult a physician for any health issues and always seek the advice of a physician before modifying diet, supplement, or exercise regimens.*

The author and publisher shall have neither liability nor responsibility to any person or entity concerning any loss or damage related to the information contained in this book. The information provided is general in nature and may not apply to every individual. Any reliance on the information contained herein is solely at the reader's own risk.

Contents

Introduction

Cardiac arrest is one of the few emergencies that demand immediate and decisive action. When the heart stops beating and a patient loses consciousness, every passing minute without blood flow causes damage to vital organs, including the heart and brain. The window of opportunity for bringing a patient back from the brink of death is small. Administering proper cardiopulmonary resuscitation (CPR) can be the difference between life and death.

This book provides instructions for mastering the core techniques of CPR to help save lives. When cardiac arrest strikes, knowledge of how to quickly open airways, restore oxygen, provide chest compressions, and use electrical therapies can make all the difference. Effective CPR circulates blood until the heart can resume a normal rhythm or pace. Skills covered range from basic CPR everyone should know to advanced interventions for medical providers.

Inside, you will learn CPR methods that conform to the latest consensus guidelines. Topics span recognizing cardiac arrest, performing high-quality chest compressions, properly administering ventilation, operating automated external defibrillators (AEDs), and providing post-resuscitation care.

Special techniques for infants, children, pregnant patients, and cases involving drowning, trauma, or poisoning are also covered. Whether you are a layperson, lifeguard, EMT, nurse, or physician, mastering these techniques will prepare you to take decisive lifesaving actions in emergencies.

When seconds count in resuscitating unresponsive patients, this definitive guide provides CPR knowledge that can make the difference between life and death. Equipped with these techniques, you gain the power to help restart the heartbeat of life when it matters most.

Chapter 1

Understanding Cardiopulmonary Resuscitation (CPR)

What is Cardiopulmonary Resuscitation (CPR)?

Cardiopulmonary resuscitation, commonly known as CPR, is a life-saving technique used to revive individuals who have experienced cardiac arrest or stopped breathing. Performing CPR is a crucial skill that anyone can learn, regardless of their medical knowledge. In this section, we will explore the fundamental aspects of CPR, including its purpose, the basic steps involved, and the significance of early intervention.

The Purpose of CPR

The primary goal of CPR is to maintain blood flow and oxygenation to vital organs, particularly the brain, and heart, when the body's natural circulation and breathing have ceased. By performing CPR, you are essentially acting as the person's heart and lungs, providing the necessary oxygen and blood flow until professional medical help arrives.

The Basic Steps of CPR

CPR consists of a series of steps that should be followed in a specific order. These steps are designed to maximize the chances of survival for the individual in need. The basic steps of CPR include:

1. **Assessing the situation:** Before performing CPR, ensure the safety of yourself and others by checking for potential hazards.

2. **Checking for responsiveness:** Gently tap the person and ask loudly, "Are you okay?" If there is no response, it indicates that the person is unresponsive and requires immediate medical attention.

3. **Activating emergency medical services (EMS):** Call for help by dialing the emergency number in your country, such as 911. Provide clear and concise information about the situation, including the location and the person's condition.

4. **Performing chest compressions:** To perform chest compressions, first place the heel of one hand in the center of the person's chest, between the nipples. Interlock your fingers and ensure that your shoulders are directly above your hands. Push hard and fast, aiming for a depth of at least 2 inches (5 centimeters) and a rate of 100–120 compressions per minute. Remember to allow the chest to fully recoil between compressions.

5. **Providing rescue breaths:** After 30 compressions, open the person's airway by tilting their head back and lifting their chin. Place your hand over the person's mouth and pinch their nose closed. Give two breaths, each lasting one second, and watch their chest rise.

6. **Continuing cycles of compressions and breaths:** Repeat the cycle of 30 compressions followed by two rescue breaths until professional help arrives or the person shows signs of life.

The Importance of Early Intervention

Time is of the essence when it comes to CPR. The chances of survival decrease rapidly with each passing minute, without intervention. Performing CPR immediately after cardiac arrest significantly increases the likelihood of a positive outcome. By starting CPR promptly, you are buying valuable time for the person until advanced medical care can be provided.

The Role of CPR in the Chain of Survival

CPR is a vital link in the chain of survival, a sequence of actions that, when performed promptly, can greatly improve the chances of survival for someone experiencing cardiac arrest. The chain of survival includes four key components:

1. **Early recognition and activation:** Recognizing the signs of cardiac arrest and activating the emergency response system promptly.

2. **Early CPR:** Initiating CPR immediately to maintain blood flow and oxygenation to vital organs.
3. **Early defibrillation:** Using an automated external defibrillator (AED) to deliver an electric shock to the heart, if available.
4. **Early advanced care:** Receiving advanced medical care from healthcare professionals, such as paramedics or doctors, as soon as possible.

Each link in the chain is essential, and the success of CPR relies on the seamless coordination of these components. By understanding and implementing CPR effectively, you become an integral part of the chain of survival, increasing the chances of a positive outcome for the person in need.

The Importance of CPR in Saving Lives

Cardiopulmonary resuscitation (CPR) is a life-saving technique that can make a crucial difference in the outcome of a cardiac arrest or other medical emergencies. When someone's heart stops beating or they stop breathing, every second counts.

CPR provides immediate assistance to maintain blood flow and oxygenation to vital organs until professional medical help arrives. In this section, we will explore the importance of CPR in saving lives and why everyone should have a basic understanding of this technique.

The Chain of Survival

To understand the significance of CPR, it is essential to grasp the concept of the "Chain of Survival." The Chain of Survival is a series of critical steps that, when followed promptly and effectively, can greatly increase the chances of survival for a person experiencing cardiac arrest. These steps include early recognition of the emergency, early activation of emergency medical services (EMS), early CPR, and early defibrillation, followed by advanced medical care.

CPR plays a vital role in the chain of survival by maintaining blood circulation and oxygenation to the brain and other vital organs. When the heart stops beating, the brain begins to suffer from oxygen deprivation within minutes. By performing CPR, you can help circulate oxygen-rich blood to the brain and prevent irreversible brain damage.

Immediate Response

One of the key reasons why CPR is so important is that it provides an immediate response to a life-threatening situation. In cardiac arrest cases, every minute without CPR decreases the chances of survival by 7–10%. This means that if CPR is not initiated within the first few minutes, the chances of survival diminish rapidly.

By learning CPR, you become equipped to respond quickly and effectively in emergencies. You can be the difference between life and death for someone in need. Whether it's a family member, a friend, or a stranger, your knowledge of CPR can make a significant impact on their chances of survival.

Availability and Accessibility

Another crucial aspect of CPR's importance is its availability and accessibility. Cardiac arrests can happen anywhere, at any time, and to anyone. They can occur in homes, workplaces, public spaces, or even on the street. In such situations, the immediate availability of someone trained in CPR can be the determining factor in saving a life.

By learning CPR, you become part of a network of individuals who are prepared to respond to emergencies. You can be the person who steps forward and takes action when someone collapses or stops breathing. Your knowledge and skills can bridge the gap between the occurrence of a cardiac arrest and the arrival of professional medical help.

Empowerment and Confidence

Knowing how to perform CPR not only empowers you to save lives but also instills confidence in your ability to handle emergencies. In times of crisis, people often feel helpless and overwhelmed. However, with CPR training, you gain the knowledge and skills necessary to take control of the situation and provide life-saving assistance.

By being confident in your ability to perform CPR, you can remain calm and composed during emergencies. This composure can have a positive impact on the victim as well, as they may feel reassured and supported during a distressing time. Your confidence can inspire others to take action and potentially save more lives.

Public Health Impact

CPR is not just about individual life-saving; it also has a broader public health impact. When more people in a community are trained in CPR, the chances of survival for cardiac arrest victims increase significantly. By spreading awareness and knowledge about CPR, we can create a society where more lives are saved.

Furthermore, CPR training can also help prevent unnecessary deaths due to choking or drowning incidents. By understanding the techniques and steps involved in CPR, individuals can respond promptly and effectively in various emergencies.

The History and Evolution of CPR

Cardiopulmonary resuscitation, commonly known as CPR, has a rich history that spans centuries. The techniques and methods used in CPR have evolved significantly over time, leading to improved outcomes and increased survival rates. In this section, we will explore the fascinating journey of CPR, from its humble beginnings to the advanced life-saving techniques used today.

Early Beginnings

The roots of CPR can be traced back to ancient civilizations. As early as 3000 BCE, the ancient Egyptians depicted scenes of chest compressions on their hieroglyphs, suggesting a rudimentary understanding of the importance of chest compressions in reviving a person. Similarly, ancient Chinese texts from the 11th century described a technique called "the method of blowing air into the mouth" to resuscitate drowning victims.

The Renaissance and the Birth of Modern CPR

During the Renaissance period, medical knowledge and practices began to advance significantly. In the 16th century, Andreas Vesalius, a Belgian anatomist, conducted groundbreaking research on the human body, including the heart and lungs. His work laid the foundation for a better understanding of the cardiovascular system and the importance of circulation in maintaining life.

In the 18th century, the concept of artificial respiration emerged. The Paris Academy of Sciences recommended the use of mouth-to-mouth resuscitation, which involved blowing air into the victim's mouth, as a method to revive drowning victims. This technique was further refined in the 19th century by Dr. Henry Silvester, who introduced the Silvester Method of artificial respiration. This method involved raising and lowering the arms alternately to facilitate breathing.

The Birth of Modern CPR

The modern era of CPR began in the early 1960s, when Dr. James Elam and Dr. Peter Safar independently discovered the effectiveness of mouth-to-mouth resuscitation combined with chest compressions. Their research showed that the combination of these techniques could maintain blood flow and oxygenation, increasing the chances of survival.

In 1960, the American Heart Association (AHA) recognized the potential of CPR and established the CPR Committee. This committee was responsible for developing standardized guidelines and training programs to teach CPR to the general public. The AHA's efforts were instrumental in popularizing CPR and making it accessible to everyone.

The Introduction of External Defibrillation

In the 1980s, the introduction of external defibrillation revolutionized the field of CPR. Defibrillation is the process of delivering an electric shock to the heart to restore its normal rhythm. The development of automated external defibrillators (AEDs) has made defibrillation more accessible and user-friendly. AEDs are now widely available in public places, such as airports, shopping malls, and schools, enabling bystanders to provide immediate defibrillation to cardiac arrest victims.

Continuous Chest Compressions and Hands-Only CPR

In recent years, there has been a shift towards simplifying CPR techniques to increase bystander participation and improve outcomes. Research has shown that continuous chest compressions, without interruption for rescue breaths, can be just as effective as traditional CPR with rescue breaths. This led to the development of Hands-Only CPR, which involves performing uninterrupted chest compressions at a rate of 100–120 compressions per minute.

Hands-Only CPR has gained popularity due to its simplicity and ease of use. It eliminates the hesitation that some bystanders may have in providing rescue breaths and focuses on the most critical aspect of CPR – maintaining blood flow to the vital organs.

Advancements in Training and Technology

Over the years, CPR training programs have become more accessible and comprehensive. Today, individuals can receive CPR training through various channels, including in-person classes, online courses, and mobile applications. These training programs not only teach the techniques of CPR but also provide valuable information on recognizing cardiac arrest, activating emergency medical services, and using AEDs.

Technological advancements have also played a significant role in improving CPR outcomes. Feedback devices, such as

CPR manikins with built-in sensors, provide real-time feedback on the quality of chest compressions, ensuring that rescuers maintain the correct depth and rate. These devices help individuals gain confidence in their CPR skills and improve the effectiveness of their interventions.

The history and evolution of CPR have been marked by significant milestones and advancements. From ancient civilizations to modern-day techniques, CPR has come a long way in saving lives.

The continuous efforts of medical professionals, researchers, and organizations like the American Heart Association have contributed to the widespread adoption of CPR and increased survival rates. As we continue to learn and innovate, CPR will undoubtedly evolve further, ensuring that more lives are saved in the future.

Common Misconceptions about CPR

Cardiopulmonary resuscitation (CPR) is a life-saving technique that can significantly increase the chances of survival for someone experiencing cardiac arrest. However, several common misconceptions about CPR can hinder its effectiveness and potentially put lives at risk. In this section, we will address these misconceptions and provide accurate information to help you better understand and perform CPR.

Misconception 1: *CPR is only necessary for older adults.*
One of the most prevalent misconceptions about CPR is that it is only needed for older adults. In reality, cardiac arrest can occur at any age, including infants, children, and young adults. It is crucial to remember that CPR is not limited to a specific age group. By being prepared and knowledgeable about CPR techniques, you can potentially save a life, regardless of the person's age.

Misconception 2: *CPR always results in a successful revival.*
While CPR is a vital intervention during cardiac arrest, it does not guarantee a successful revival in every case. The purpose of CPR is to maintain blood flow and oxygenation to vital organs until advanced medical help arrives. The outcome of CPR depends on various factors, including the underlying cause of cardiac arrest, the timeliness of CPR initiation, and the availability of advanced medical care. It is essential to understand that CPR is not a guaranteed solution but rather a critical step in the chain of survival.

Misconception 3: *CPR can restart a stopped heart.*
Another common misconception is that CPR can restart a stopped heart. In reality, CPR helps to circulate oxygenated blood to vital organs, including the brain, during cardiac arrest. It does not directly restart the heart. The objective of CPR is to buy time until a defibrillator or advanced medical care can be administered to restore the heart's normal rhythm.

CPR is a crucial bridge to more advanced interventions, such as defibrillation, which can potentially restart the heart.

Misconception 4: *Mouth-to-mouth resuscitation is always necessary.*

Many people believe that mouth-to-mouth resuscitation is always required during CPR. However, the guidelines for CPR have evolved, and the emphasis is now primarily on high-quality chest compressions. In most cases, hands-only CPR, which involves uninterrupted chest compressions, is sufficient until professional help arrives. Mouth-to-mouth resuscitation may still be necessary in certain situations, such as drowning incidents, or when the rescuer is trained and comfortable performing it.

Misconception 5: *CPR is dangerous and can cause harm.*

Some individuals may hesitate to perform CPR due to the fear of causing harm. However, the risks associated with performing CPR are minimal compared to the potential benefits of saving a life. The American Heart Association (AHA) and other reputable organizations provide guidelines and training to ensure that CPR is performed safely and effectively. Remember, any attempt at CPR is better than no attempt at all, as it can significantly increase the chances of survival for someone in cardiac arrest.

Misconception 6: *CPR is only effective if performed by healthcare professionals.*

While healthcare professionals receive extensive training in CPR, it is not limited to their expertise. Bystander CPR, performed by individuals who are not healthcare professionals, has been shown to significantly improve survival rates for cardiac arrest victims. Prompt initiation of CPR by anyone present at the scene can make a crucial difference in the outcome. It is important to remember that even if you are not a healthcare professional, you can still learn and perform CPR effectively.

Misconception 7: *CPR is no longer necessary if the person shows signs of life.*

Another misconception is that CPR is no longer necessary if the person shows signs of life, such as coughing or gasping. These signs, known as agonal breathing, are not indicative of normal breathing and should not be mistaken for signs of recovery. Agonal breathing is a reflexive response of the brainstem and does not provide sufficient oxygenation to sustain life. CPR should be continued until professional help arrives and takes over the resuscitation efforts.

Misconception 8: *CPR is only effective in a hospital setting.*

CPR is not limited to a hospital setting and can be performed effectively in various environments, including homes, workplaces, and public spaces. The majority of cardiac arrests occur outside of hospitals. Immediate initiation of CPR by bystanders can significantly improve the chances of survival before emergency medical services arrive. It is crucial to be prepared and confident in performing CPR wherever and whenever it is needed.

Misconception 9: *A pulse check is necessary before starting CPR.*

Traditionally, a pulse check was recommended before starting CPR. However, recent guidelines emphasize the importance of starting CPR immediately if the person is unresponsive and not breathing normally. In high-stress situations, it can be challenging to accurately detect a pulse, leading to unnecessary delays in starting CPR. Therefore, the focus now is on recognizing the absence of normal breathing and promptly initiating CPR.

Misconception 10: *CPR is a complex technique that requires extensive training.*

While formal CPR training is highly recommended, it is not a prerequisite for performing CPR. The basic principles of CPR, such as chest compressions and rescue breaths, can be learned quickly and easily. Many organizations offer CPR courses and certifications that provide hands-on training and practice. However, even without formal training, performing hands-only CPR can still make a significant difference in saving a life. Remember, any attempt at CPR is better than no attempt at all.

By dispelling these common misconceptions about CPR, we hope to empower you with accurate knowledge and encourage you to take action in emergencies. CPR is a critical skill that can save lives, and by understanding its principles and techniques, you can become a valuable link in the chain of survival.

Chapter 2

Preparing for CPR

Assessing the Situation and Ensuring Safety

When faced with a medical emergency, every second counts. The first step in preparing for cardiopulmonary resuscitation (CPR) is to assess the situation and ensure the safety of both yourself and the victim. This crucial step sets the foundation for a successful resuscitation attempt and can make a significant difference in saving a life.

Assessing the Situation

Before jumping into action, take a moment to assess the situation. Look around and evaluate the environment for any potential hazards or dangers that could pose a threat to you or the victim. This assessment is essential to ensuring your safety and the safety of others present.

Start by checking for any immediate dangers, such as traffic, fire, or falling objects. If necessary, move the victim to a safer location away from these hazards. Remember, your safety should always be a priority, and you cannot help the victim if you become injured or put yourself in harm's way.

Next, evaluate the victim's condition. Determine if they are conscious or unconscious. If the victim is conscious, ask them simple questions to assess their mental state and level of awareness. If they are unable to respond or their responses are incoherent, it may indicate a more severe medical emergency.

If the victim is unconscious, check for signs of breathing. Look for chest rise and fall, listen for any sounds of breathing, and feel for air movement on your cheek. If the victim is not breathing or only gasping, it is a clear indication of cardiac arrest, and immediate CPR is necessary.

Ensuring Safety

Once you have assessed the situation and determined the need for CPR, it is crucial to ensure the safety of both yourself and the victim throughout the resuscitation process. By following a few simple guidelines, you can minimize risks and maximize the chances of a successful outcome.

First and foremost, make sure you have protective gloves available. Gloves not only protect you from potential infections but also provide a barrier between you and the victim's bodily fluids. In an emergency situation, it is essential to prioritize your safety and take precautions to prevent the spread of diseases.

If possible, ask someone nearby to call emergency medical services (EMS) while you begin CPR. Promptly activating

EMS ensures that professional help is on the way and can provide additional support and advanced medical care upon their arrival.

When performing CPR, position yourself correctly to maintain stability and maximize the effectiveness of your compressions. Kneel beside the victim's chest, aligning your shoulders directly above your hands. This position allows you to use your upper-body strength efficiently and deliver effective chest compressions.

Remember to remove any clothing or objects that may interfere with CPR. Open the victim's airway by tilting their head back and lifting their chin. This maneuver helps to clear any obstructions and allows for better airflow during rescue breaths.

While performing CPR, it is crucial to maintain a steady rhythm and depth with your compressions. Aim for a compression depth of at least two inches for adults and children and about 1.5 inches for infants. Ensure that you allow the chest to fully recoil between compressions to facilitate blood flow.

In situations where an automated external defibrillator (AED) is available, follow the device's instructions carefully. AEDs are designed to analyze the victim's heart rhythm and deliver a shock if necessary. Make sure the victim's chest is dry before attaching the AED pads, and avoid touching the victim during the analysis and shock delivery.

It is critical to communicate properly with any spectators or other individuals present throughout the resuscitation process. Assign specific tasks to individuals around you, such as calling for assistance, fetching more equipment, or offering emotional support. Everyone is on the same page and working together to save the victim's life when there is clear communication.

Assessing the situation and ensuring safety are critical steps in preparing for CPR. By evaluating the environment for potential hazards and taking necessary precautions, you can create a safe and effective resuscitation environment. Remember to prioritize your safety and the safety of others while providing life-saving care.

Activating Emergency Medical Services (EMS)

When faced with a medical emergency, time is of the essence. Activating Emergency Medical Services (EMS) is a crucial step in the chain of survival. EMS consists of a team of highly trained professionals who are equipped to provide immediate medical assistance and transport patients to the nearest healthcare facility. In this section, we will discuss the importance of activating EMS, how to do it effectively, and the information you need to provide.

Why is Activating EMS Important?

Activating EMS is vital because it ensures that professional medical help is on its way while you are performing CPR. EMS personnel are trained to handle emergencies and have access to advanced medical equipment and resources that can significantly improve the chances of survival for the patient.

By activating EMS, you are also initiating a coordinated response system that involves paramedics, emergency medical technicians (EMTs), and other healthcare professionals. These individuals are trained to assess the situation, provide immediate medical interventions, and transport the patient to the appropriate healthcare facility for further treatment.

How to Activate EMS

Activating EMS should be done as quickly as possible, ideally before starting CPR. Here are the steps to follow:

1. **Assess the situation:** Before activating EMS, assess the scene for any potential dangers or hazards. Ensure your safety and the safety of others before proceeding.
2. **Dial the emergency number:** In most countries, the emergency number is 911. Dial this number to connect with the emergency dispatch center. If you are in a different country, familiarize yourself with the local emergency number.
3. **Provide accurate information:** When speaking to the emergency dispatcher, remain calm and provide

accurate information about the situation. Be prepared to answer questions such as the location of the emergency, the nature of the problem, and the number of individuals requiring assistance.

4. **Follow the dispatcher's instructions:** The dispatcher may provide you with instructions on how to perform CPR or other life-saving interventions until EMS arrives. Follow their guidance carefully.

5. **Stay on the line:** Do not hang up until the dispatcher tells you to do so. They may need additional information or provide further instructions.

Information to Provide to EMS

When activating EMS, it is essential to provide accurate and concise information to ensure a prompt and appropriate response. Here are the key details you should provide:

1. **Location:** Clearly state the address or location of the emergency. If you are unsure of the exact address, provide landmarks or any other identifiable information that can help EMS locate you quickly.

2. **Nature of the emergency:** Describe the situation briefly and clearly. For example, if someone is experiencing cardiac arrest, state that the person is unresponsive and not breathing.

3. **Number of individuals involved:** If there are multiple victims, inform the dispatcher about the total number

of individuals requiring assistance. This information helps EMS allocate appropriate resources.

4. **Any special circumstances:** If any unique circumstances may affect the response, such as hazardous materials or difficult access to the location, inform the dispatcher.

Remember, the more accurate and detailed information you provide, the better equipped EMS will be to respond effectively.

Additional Considerations

While activating EMS is crucial, there are a few additional considerations to keep in mind:

1. **Stay with the patient:** If possible, assign someone to stay with the patient while you activate EMS. This ensures that CPR or other life-saving interventions can continue until professional help arrives.

2. **Follow local protocols:** Different regions may have specific protocols for activating EMS. Familiarize yourself with the guidelines and procedures in your area to ensure a seamless response.

3. **Stay calm and focused:** During a medical emergency, it is natural to feel overwhelmed. However, it is essential to remain calm and focused while activating EMS. Clear communication and accurate information are vital for a successful response.

4. **Be prepared to provide updates:** If the patient's condition changes or if there are any significant developments, update the dispatcher accordingly. This information helps EMS adjust their response and provide appropriate care.

Remember, activating EMS is a critical step in the chain of survival. By promptly alerting professional medical help, you are increasing the chances of a positive outcome for the patient.

Gathering and Using Available Resources

When faced with a cardiac arrest situation, it is crucial to gather and utilize all available resources effectively. The success of cardiopulmonary resuscitation (CPR) relies not only on your skills and knowledge but also on the tools and support systems you have at your disposal. In this section, we will explore the various resources you can gather and how to use them efficiently to maximize the chances of saving a life.

Assessing the Situation

Before you begin CPR, it is essential to assess the situation and gather information about the victim's condition. Look for any signs of responsiveness or breathing. If the victim is unresponsive and not breathing or only gasping, it is likely a cardiac arrest situation. Quickly determine if any bystanders can assist you. Assign specific tasks to them, such as calling emergency medical services (EMS) or retrieving an automated external defibrillator (AED).

Activating Emergency Medical Services (EMS)

One of the most critical resources in a cardiac arrest situation is EMS. As soon as you recognize the need for CPR, it is crucial to activate EMS by calling the emergency number in your country. Provide them with accurate information about the victim's condition and location. Stay on the line with the dispatcher, as they can provide guidance and support until help arrives.

Bystander Assistance

Bystanders can be valuable resources during a cardiac arrest emergency. They can help you gather additional resources and provide support. Assign specific tasks to bystanders, such as calling EMS, retrieving an AED, or finding a first aid kit. Communicate instructions and ensure that they understand their roles. Bystanders can also offer emotional support to the victim's family or provide crowd control if necessary.

Automated External Defibrillators (AEDs)

AEDs are portable devices that can analyze a person's heart rhythm and deliver an electric shock if necessary. These devices are crucial in restoring a normal heart rhythm during a cardiac arrest. Many public places, such as airports, shopping malls, and schools, have AEDs readily available. If an AED is nearby, instruct a bystander to retrieve it while you continue with CPR. Follow the AED's voice prompts and apply the pads to the victim's chest as directed. AEDs are designed to be user-friendly, and they provide clear instructions on how to proceed.

First Aid Kits

First aid kits contain essential supplies that can be useful in a cardiac arrest situation. While CPR primarily focuses on chest compressions and rescue breaths, having access to a first aid kit can be beneficial. These kits typically include items such as gloves, bandages, and antiseptic wipes. They can be used to address any injuries or wounds that may have contributed to the cardiac arrest or occurred during the resuscitation process.

Personal Protective Equipment (PPE)

When performing CPR, it is crucial to protect yourself and others from potential risks, such as bloodborne pathogens. Personal protective equipment (PPE) includes gloves, masks, and face shields. These items create a barrier between you and the victim, reducing the risk of infection transmission. Ensure that you have access to PPE and use it appropriately to maintain a safe environment for everyone involved.

Communication Devices

Effective communication is vital during a cardiac arrest emergency. Having access to communication devices, such as mobile phones or two-way radios, can help you coordinate with EMS, bystanders, or other healthcare professionals.

These devices allow you to provide updates, receive instructions, or seek additional assistance if needed. Make sure your communication devices are fully charged and easily accessible during emergencies.

Training and Education Materials

Continuous learning and staying updated on CPR techniques and guidelines are essential for providing high-quality resuscitation. Gather and utilize training and education materials to enhance your knowledge and skills. These resources can include books, online courses, videos, or workshops. Stay informed about the latest advancements in CPR and regularly practice your skills to maintain proficiency.

Support from Healthcare Professionals

In some situations, you may need additional support from healthcare professionals. This can include paramedics, nurses, or doctors who can provide advanced medical interventions or guidance during the resuscitation process. If available, seek their assistance and collaborate with them to ensure the best possible outcome for the victim.

Psychological Support

Performing CPR can be emotionally challenging, especially if the outcome is not favorable. It is essential to have access to psychological support resources for both yourself and the victim's family. This can include counseling services, support groups, or helplines. Recognize the emotional impact of performing CPR and seek support when needed.

Remember, gathering and using available resources effectively can significantly improve the chances of a successful resuscitation. Assess the situation, activate EMS, utilize bystander assistance, and make use of tools such as AEDs and first aid kits.

Protect yourself with PPE, communicate effectively with the help of communication devices, and continuously educate yourself through training materials. Seek support from healthcare professionals and psychological resources to cope with the emotional aspects of CPR. By utilizing these resources, you can become a more effective lifesaver and increase the likelihood of saving lives.

Understanding Legal and Ethical Considerations

When it comes to performing cardiopulmonary resuscitation (CPR), it is essential to not only understand the life-saving techniques but also the legal and ethical considerations that surround this critical intervention. In this section, we will explore the legal protections, ethical obligations, and potential challenges that individuals may encounter when performing CPR.

Legal Protections for CPR Providers

In many jurisdictions, there are legal protections in place to encourage individuals to provide CPR without fear of liability. These protections are commonly known as Good Samaritan laws. Good Samaritan laws vary from country to country and even from state to state, so it is important to familiarize yourself with the specific laws in your area.

Good Samaritan laws generally provide legal immunity to individuals who provide CPR in good faith and without expectation of compensation. These laws are designed to encourage bystanders to intervene in emergencies without hesitation. However, it is important to note that these laws do not protect individuals from gross negligence or intentional harm.

To ensure you are protected under Good Samaritan laws, it is crucial to act within your level of training and competence. If you have received CPR certification, it is important to adhere to the guidelines and techniques taught during your training. By following these guidelines, you can demonstrate that you acted in good faith and within the scope of your training.

Ethical Considerations in CPR

While legal protections provide some reassurance, it is equally important to consider the ethical implications of performing CPR. Ethical considerations revolve around the principles of beneficence, autonomy, and justice.

Beneficence refers to the duty to do good and act in the best interest of the patient. When faced with a cardiac arrest situation, providing CPR is generally considered the morally right thing to do. By initiating CPR, you are attempting to restore blood circulation and oxygenation, giving the individual a chance at survival.

Autonomy, on the other hand, recognizes an individual's right to make decisions about their own healthcare. In some cases, individuals may have expressed their wishes to not receive CPR through advance directives or do-not-resuscitate (DNR) orders. It is crucial to respect these wishes and honor their autonomy. However, in the absence of such directives, it is generally assumed that individuals would want life-saving measures to be taken.

Justice plays a role in ensuring fair and equal access to CPR. It is important to provide CPR to anyone in need, regardless of their age, gender, race, or socioeconomic status. Every individual deserves an equal chance at survival, and withholding CPR based on discriminatory factors is ethically unacceptable.

Challenges and Ethical Dilemmas

While the legal and ethical frameworks surrounding CPR provide guidance, there can still be challenges and ethical dilemmas that arise in real-life situations. One common challenge is the uncertainty of a person's wishes regarding

CPR. In some cases, individuals may not have expressed their preferences through advance directives or DNR orders, leaving healthcare providers and bystanders unsure of the appropriate course of action. In such situations, it is crucial to err on the side of providing CPR, as it is generally considered the default action in the absence of clear instructions.

Another challenge is the emotional toll that performing CPR can have on individuals. CPR can be physically demanding and emotionally distressing, especially if the outcome is not favorable. CPR providers need to have access to emotional support and debriefing after performing CPR to process their experiences and cope with any emotional distress that may arise.

Additionally, cultural and religious beliefs may influence an individual's perspective on CPR. Some cultures or religions may have specific beliefs or practices regarding end-of-life care, which may conflict with the standard CPR protocols. It is important to respect and consider these beliefs while providing CPR, if possible, without compromising the individual's chances of survival.

Understanding the legal and ethical considerations surrounding CPR is crucial for anyone involved in providing this life-saving intervention. Good Samaritan laws provide legal protections, while ethical principles guide decision-making in CPR situations. By being aware of these considerations, individuals can confidently and responsibly perform CPR, potentially saving lives in the process.

Chapter 3

Basic Life Support (BLS)

Recognizing Cardiac Arrest and Performing the Chain of Survival

Cardiac arrest is a life-threatening emergency that occurs when the heart suddenly stops beating. It is crucial to recognize the signs of cardiac arrest promptly and initiate the chain of survival to increase the chances of saving a person's life. In this section, we will discuss how to recognize cardiac arrest and the steps involved in performing the chain of survival.

Recognizing Cardiac Arrest

Recognizing cardiac arrest is the first step in providing timely and effective cardiopulmonary resuscitation (CPR). It is essential to be aware of the common signs and symptoms of cardiac arrest, which include:

1. **Sudden loss of responsiveness:** The person becomes unresponsive and does not react to any stimuli, such as shaking or shouting.

2. **Absence of normal breathing:** The person stops breathing or only gasps irregularly. Gasping is not considered normal breathing and is often a sign of cardiac arrest.

3. **No pulse or signs of circulation:** Check for a pulse at the carotid artery (neck) or the brachial artery (wrist). If there is no pulse or signs of circulation, it indicates cardiac arrest.

Remember, recognizing cardiac arrest is crucial, as immediate action can significantly improve the chances of survival. If you suspect someone is experiencing cardiac arrest, it is essential to act quickly and initiate the chain of survival.

The Chain of Survival

The chain of survival is a series of critical steps that, when performed promptly and effectively, can greatly increase the chances of survival for a person experiencing cardiac arrest. The chain of survival consists of four key links:

1. **Early recognition and activation:** As mentioned earlier, recognizing cardiac arrest promptly is crucial. If you witness someone collapse or find an unresponsive person, immediately activate the emergency response system by calling for help or asking someone nearby to call emergency medical services (EMS). Time is of the essence, and the sooner help arrives, the better the chances of survival.

2. **Early CPR:** Cardiopulmonary resuscitation (CPR) is a vital component of the chain of survival. If you are trained in CPR, begin chest compressions immediately after recognizing cardiac arrest. High-quality chest compressions help circulate oxygenated blood to vital organs, including the brain until advanced medical help arrives.

3. **Early defibrillation:** Defibrillation is the delivery of an electric shock to the heart to restore its normal rhythm. Automated external defibrillators (AEDs) are portable devices that can analyze the heart's rhythm and deliver a shock if necessary. If an AED is available, it should be used as soon as possible. Early defibrillation significantly improves the chances of restoring a normal heart rhythm.

4. **Early advanced care:** Advanced medical care provided by healthcare professionals, such as paramedics or emergency room physicians, is crucial for the successful resuscitation of a person in cardiac arrest. These professionals have the skills and equipment necessary to provide advanced cardiac life support (ACLS) and further interventions to stabilize the person's condition.

Remember, each link in the chain of survival is essential, and the success of resuscitation depends on the seamless integration of these steps. By recognizing cardiac arrest promptly and initiating the chain of survival, you can play a vital role in saving a person's life.

Importance of Early Intervention

Early intervention is critical in cardiac arrest cases because the longer the delay in initiating CPR and defibrillation, the lower the chances of survival. Research has shown that for every minute that passes without CPR and defibrillation, the chances of survival decrease by approximately 7–10%.

By recognizing cardiac arrest promptly and starting CPR immediately, you can help maintain blood flow to vital organs and increase the likelihood of a successful resuscitation. CPR provides oxygen to the brain and other organs, preventing irreversible damage until advanced medical care can be provided.

Additionally, early defibrillation is crucial in cases where the cardiac arrest is caused by a specific type of abnormal heart rhythm called ventricular fibrillation (VF) or ventricular tachycardia (VT). These rhythms can often be corrected by delivering a shock through an AED, restoring the heart's normal rhythm and increasing the chances of survival.

Recognizing cardiac arrest and performing the chain of survival are fundamental skills in mastering cardiopulmonary resuscitation. By being able to identify the signs of cardiac arrest and initiating the chain of survival promptly, you can significantly increase the chances of saving a person's life. Remember, every second counts, and your actions can make a difference in someone's survival. In the next section, we will delve into the specifics of performing high-quality chest compressions.

Performing High-Quality Chest Compressions

Performing high-quality chest compressions is a critical component of basic life support (BLS) and can greatly increase the chances of survival for someone experiencing cardiac arrest. In this section, we will explore the key principles and techniques for delivering effective chest compressions.

The Importance of Chest Compressions

During cardiac arrest, the heart stops pumping blood effectively, depriving the body of oxygen. Chest compressions help to manually circulate blood to vital organs, including the brain until advanced medical help arrives. By compressing the chest, you are essentially acting as the heart, maintaining blood flow and increasing the likelihood of a successful resuscitation.

Positioning and Technique

To perform high-quality chest compressions, it is important to position yourself correctly and use the proper technique. Follow these steps:

1. **Positioning:** Place the person on a firm, flat surface. Kneel beside them, ensuring that their chest is at the same level as your hands. This will allow you to apply adequate pressure during compressions.

2. **Hand Placement:** Position the heel of one hand on the center of the person's chest, between the nipples. Place your other hand on top, interlocking your fingers. Ensure that your fingers are lifted off the chest to avoid interfering with the compressions.

3. **Compression Depth:** Press down firmly and quickly, aiming for a compression depth of at least 2 inches (5 centimeters) for adults. Remember, the goal is to compress the chest enough to create blood flow without causing unnecessary harm.

4. **Compression Rate:** Aim for a compression rate of 100 to 120 compressions per minute. This equates to roughly 2 compressions per second. To maintain an appropriate rate, you can mentally count "one and two and three and four" or use a metronome if available.

5. **Allowing Full Recoil:** After each compression, allow the chest to fully recoil. This means letting it return to its normal position before starting the next compression. Allowing full recoil ensures that blood can flow back into the heart, ready for the next compression.

6. **Minimizing Interruptions:** Try to minimize interruptions in chest compressions as much as possible. Interruptions can decrease the effectiveness of CPR and reduce the chances of a successful outcome. If you need to switch with another rescuer, do so quickly and smoothly without delaying compressions.

Monitoring Compression Quality

It is crucial to monitor the quality of your chest compressions to ensure they are effective. Here are some key points to keep in mind:

1. **Depth:** Check the depth of your compressions regularly. If you find that your compressions are too shallow, adjust your technique to achieve the recommended depth of at least 2 inches (5 centimeters).

2. **Rate:** Continuously monitor your compression rate to ensure it falls within the recommended range of 100 to 120 compressions per minute. If you find yourself going too fast or too slow, make the necessary adjustments.

3. **Allowing Full Recoil:** Pay attention to the recoil of the chest after each compression. Make sure you are allowing the chest to fully recoil before starting the next compression. This will ensure optimal blood flow.

4. **Minimizing Fatigue:** Performing chest compressions can be physically demanding, and rescuers may experience fatigue over time. If you notice a decline in the quality of your compressions due to fatigue, switch with another rescuer if possible.

Challenges and Troubleshooting

Performing high-quality chest compressions can be challenging, especially in high-stress situations. Here are some common challenges you may encounter and how to troubleshoot them:

1. **Fatigue:** As mentioned earlier, fatigue can affect the quality of your compressions. If you feel tired, switch with another rescuer to maintain the effectiveness of CPR.

2. **Inadequate Depth:** If you find that your compressions are consistently too shallow, adjust your technique and apply more pressure to achieve the recommended depth.

3. **Compression Rate Variations:** It is common for rescuers to deviate from the recommended compression rate. If you notice that you are going too fast or too slow, focus on maintaining a steady rhythm and adjust your pace accordingly.

4. **Rib Fractures:** In some cases, the force applied during chest compressions may result in rib fractures. While

this is an unfortunate side effect, it should not deter you from performing CPR. Remember, the priority is to save a life, and the benefits of chest compressions far outweigh the risks.

Continuous Training and Improvement

Performing high-quality chest compressions requires practice and ongoing training. It is essential to stay updated with the latest guidelines and techniques. Consider attending CPR courses or workshops regularly to refresh your skills and knowledge. Additionally, seek feedback from experienced healthcare professionals to improve your technique and ensure you are providing the best possible care.

Remember, your ability to perform high-quality chest compressions can make a significant difference in someone's chance of survival during a cardiac arrest. By mastering this essential skill, you become a vital link in the chain of survival, helping to save lives in critical situations.

Providing Effective Rescue Breaths

When performing cardiopulmonary resuscitation (CPR), providing effective rescue breaths is a crucial component of the resuscitation process. Rescue breaths help deliver oxygen to the lungs and vital organs of a person experiencing cardiac arrest. In this section, we will discuss the importance of rescue breaths, the technique for providing them, and some common considerations to keep in mind.

The Importance of Rescue Breaths

During cardiac arrest, the heart stops pumping blood effectively, leading to a lack of oxygen supply to the body's vital organs. Rescue breaths play a vital role in delivering oxygen to the lungs and facilitating the oxygenation of the blood. By providing rescue breaths, you are helping to maintain the oxygen supply to the brain and other organs, increasing the chances of a successful resuscitation.

The Technique for Providing Rescue Breaths

To provide effective rescue breaths, follow these steps:

1. Ensure the person is lying on their back on a firm surface.
2. Open the airway by tilting the head back and lifting the chin. This helps to clear any obstructions and allows for better airflow.
3. Pinch the person's nose closed with your thumb and index finger to prevent air from escaping.
4. Take a normal breath and place your mouth firmly over the person's mouth, creating an airtight seal.
5. Blow into the person's mouth for about one second, watching for the chest to rise. Ensure that you provide enough air to make the chest visibly rise, but avoid excessive force.
6. Remove your mouth from the person's mouth and allow the chest to fall, indicating exhalation.

7. Repeat the process, providing a total of two rescue breaths.

8. After providing the rescue breaths, resume chest compressions by placing your hands on the lower half of the person's sternum and performing compressions at a rate of 100–120 compressions per minute.

Remember, the quality of rescue breaths is essential. Ensure that you provide enough air to make the chest rise visibly, but avoid excessive force that could cause injury. It is also important to maintain a good seal over the person's mouth to prevent air leakage.

Considerations for Providing Rescue Breaths

While providing rescue breaths, there are a few considerations to keep in mind:

1. Personal Safety

Always prioritize your personal safety when providing rescue breaths. Ensure that the scene is safe and free from any potential hazards before initiating CPR. If there are any risks present, such as fire, electrical hazards, or dangerous substances, wait for the appropriate authorities to arrive and address the situation.

2. Airway Obstructions

In some cases, the person's airway may be obstructed by foreign objects, vomit, or other substances. Before providing rescue breaths, check for any visible obstructions and remove them if possible. If you encounter an obstruction that you cannot remove, perform the Heimlich maneuver or back blows to dislodge the object before continuing with rescue breaths.

3. Special Considerations for Children and Infants

When providing rescue breaths to children and infants, it is important to modify the technique slightly to accommodate their smaller airways. Instead of pinching the nose closed, cover both the nose and mouth with your mouth to create a seal. Additionally, provide gentler breaths to avoid overinflating their lungs.

4. Personal Protective Equipment (PPE)

In certain situations, such as during a pandemic or when dealing with individuals who may have contagious diseases, it is advisable to use personal protective equipment (PPE) like gloves, masks, and eye protection. This helps protect both the rescuer and the person receiving CPR.

5. Continuous Chest Compressions

In some cases, it may not be possible or safe to provide rescue breaths. In such situations, continuous chest compressions alone can still be effective in maintaining blood circulation and oxygenation. This technique, known as hands-only CPR, is particularly useful when the rescuer is untrained or uncomfortable providing rescue breaths.

Remember, the goal of CPR is to provide immediate care until professional medical help arrives. By providing effective rescue breaths, you are playing a crucial role in increasing the chances of survival for someone experiencing cardiac arrest.

Using Automated External Defibrillators (AEDs)

In this section, we will explore the importance of using Automated External Defibrillators (AEDs) in cardiopulmonary resuscitation (CPR) and how to effectively use them to save lives. AEDs are portable devices that can analyze a person's heart rhythm and deliver an electric shock if necessary to restore a normal heartbeat. They are designed to be user-friendly, even for individuals with little to no medical training.

Understanding the Role of AEDs in CPR

AEDs play a crucial role in the chain of survival during a cardiac arrest. When a person experiences a sudden cardiac arrest, their heart may enter a chaotic rhythm called ventricular fibrillation (VF) or a rapid rhythm called ventricular tachycardia (VT). These abnormal rhythms can be fatal if not corrected promptly. AEDs are specifically designed to detect these rhythms and deliver a shock to the heart to restore its normal rhythm.

The Importance of Early Defibrillation

Time is of the essence when it comes to cardiac arrest. Every minute that passes without defibrillation decreases the chances of survival by approximately 7–10%. Therefore, early defibrillation is crucial to improving the chances of a successful resuscitation. AEDs are designed to be readily available in public places, such as airports, shopping malls, and schools, to ensure that they can be accessed quickly in case of an emergency.

Using an AED: A Step-by-Step Guide

Using an AED may seem intimidating at first, but these devices are designed to guide users through the process with clear and simple instructions. Here is a step-by-step guide on how to use an AED effectively:

1. **Assess the situation:** Ensure the safety of yourself and others by checking for any potential hazards or dangers. If the person is unresponsive and not breathing normally, immediately call for emergency medical services (EMS) and retrieve the nearest AED.

2. **Power on the AED:** Once you have the AED, turn it on. Most AEDs have a prominent power button that is easily identifiable.

3. **Expose the person's chest:** Remove any clothing or obstructions from the person's chest to ensure proper electrode placement.

4. **Attach the electrode pads:** The AED will come with adhesive electrode pads. Follow the instructions on the AED to correctly place the pads on the person's bare chest. One pad should be placed on the upper right side of the chest, just below the collarbone, and the other pad on the lower left side of the chest, just above the lower ribs.

5. **Analyze the heart rhythm:** Once the electrode pads are in place, the AED will analyze the person's heart rhythm. Make sure no one is touching the person during this analysis.

6. **Follow the AED prompts:** Based on the analysis, the AED will provide voice prompts or visual instructions on whether or not to deliver a shock. If a shock is advised, ensure that no one is touching the person and press the shock button as instructed. Some AEDs may deliver the shock automatically without the need for manual activation.

7. **Perform CPR:** After delivering the shock, the AED may instruct you to perform CPR. Follow the AED's prompts and continue with high-quality chest compressions and rescue breaths until EMS arrives or the person shows signs of life.

8. **Continue to follow AED prompts:** Throughout the resuscitation process, the AED will continue to provide

prompts and instructions. It is important to follow these prompts until professional help arrives.

Safety Considerations When Using an AED

While AEDs are designed to be safe and user-friendly, it is essential to keep a few safety considerations in mind:

- Ensure that the person's chest is dry before attaching the electrode pads. If the chest is wet, dry it thoroughly to ensure proper adhesion.
- Remove any medication patches or excessive chest hair that may interfere with the electrode pad's adhesion.
- Do not touch the person or the AED while the device is analyzing the heart rhythm or delivering a shock.
- If the person is lying on a wet surface, move them to a dry area before using the AED.
- If the person has an implanted pacemaker or defibrillator, avoid placing the electrode pads directly over the device. Instead, place the pads at least one inch away from the device.

AED Maintenance and Training

To ensure the effectiveness of AEDs, regular maintenance and training are essential. AEDs should be regularly checked to ensure that they are in proper working condition. This includes checking the battery life, electrode pad expiration dates, and any necessary software updates.

Additionally, it is highly recommended to receive proper training in CPR and AED usage. Many organizations and community centers offer CPR and AED training courses, which can provide you with the knowledge and confidence to effectively respond to cardiac emergencies.

Remember, AEDs are designed to be used by anyone, regardless of their medical background. By following the simple instructions provided by the device, you can significantly increase the chances of survival for someone experiencing a cardiac arrest.

Managing Choking Emergencies

Choking is a life-threatening emergency that occurs when an object becomes lodged in the throat or windpipe, blocking the flow of air. It can happen to anyone, regardless of age or health condition. As a rescuer, knowing how to manage choking emergencies is crucial, as prompt action can save a person's life.

Recognizing Choking

The first step in managing a choking emergency is to recognize the signs of choking. The most common signs include:

1. **Inability to speak or breathe:** The person may be clutching their throat and making gasping or wheezing sounds.
2. **Panic or distress:** They may exhibit signs of anxiety, such as wide eyes or a panicked expression.
3. **Ineffective coughing:** The person may attempt to cough, but the coughs are weak or produce no sound.
4. **Bluish skin color:** If the airway is completely blocked, the person's skin may turn blue due to a lack of oxygen.

Performing the Heimlich Maneuver

The Heimlich maneuver, also known as abdominal thrusts, is a technique used to dislodge an object from a choking person's airway. Here's how to perform it:

- Stand behind the person and wrap your arms around their waist.
- Make a fist with one hand and place the thumb side against the person's abdomen, slightly above the navel and below the ribcage.
- Grasp your fist with your other hand and give quick, upward thrusts into the abdomen. Each thrust should be forceful but not excessive.
- Continue performing abdominal thrusts until the object is expelled or the person becomes unconscious.

If the person becomes unconscious, lower them gently to the ground and begin CPR immediately. Check for any visible obstructions in the mouth and remove them if possible. If you can see the object causing the obstruction, perform a finger sweep to remove it. If the object is not visible or cannot be removed, start chest compressions.

Performing Chest Compressions

When performing chest compressions on a choking person, the technique is slightly modified to account for the obstruction. Follow these steps:

- Kneel beside the person and place the heel of one hand on the center of the chest, slightly above the lower half of the breastbone.
- Place your other hand on top of the first hand and interlock your fingers.
- Position yourself directly over the person's chest and, using your body weight, push down firmly and quickly. The compression depth should be about 2 inches for adults and children and about 1.5 inches for infants.
- Perform chest compressions at a rate of 100–120 compressions per minute, allowing the chest to fully recoil between compressions.

Continue performing chest compressions until the object is expelled or medical help arrives. If, at any point, the person starts breathing normally, monitor their breathing and provide reassurance.

Performing CPR on Infants and Children

Choking emergencies can also occur in infants and children, requiring modified techniques for CPR. Here's what you need to know:

1. **For infants under 1 year old:** Perform back blows and chest thrusts instead of abdominal thrusts. Place the infant face-down on your forearm, supporting their head and neck. Deliver up to 5 back blows between the shoulder blades using the heel of your hand. If the object is still not dislodged, turn the infant face-up on a firm surface and perform up to five chest thrusts using two fingers in the center of the chest.
2. **For children over 1 year old:** Perform the Heimlich maneuver as described earlier, adjusting the force of the thrusts to the child's size and strength.

Remember, it is essential to call for emergency medical assistance as soon as possible when dealing with a choking emergency.

Preventing Choking Emergencies

Prevention is always better than cure. To reduce the risk of choking emergencies, consider the following preventive measures:

- Cut food into small, manageable pieces for young children.
- Encourage children to sit down and eat slowly, avoiding talking or laughing with a mouthful of food.
- Keep small objects, such as coins or small toys, out of reach of infants and young children.
- Avoid giving young children foods that are hard, round, or sticky, as they are more likely to cause choking.
- Educate yourself and others on proper first aid techniques, including CPR and the Heimlich maneuver.

By being prepared and knowledgeable about managing choking emergencies, you can make a significant difference in saving lives. Remember, every second counts, so act quickly and confidently when faced with a choking situation.

Special Considerations for BLS in Different Age Groups

When it comes to performing Basic Life Support (BLS), it's important to understand that different age groups may require slightly different approaches. While the core principles of BLS remain the same, certain considerations and techniques need to be taken into account when performing CPR on infants, children, and the elderly. In this section, we will explore these special considerations for BLS in different age groups.

BLS for Infants

Infants, defined as children under the age of one, have unique anatomical and physiological characteristics that require special attention during CPR. Here are some key considerations when performing BLS on infants:

1. **Positioning:** When assessing an unresponsive infant, place them on a firm surface and ensure their head is in a neutral position. Use a towel or blanket to maintain the head in a slightly extended position, ensuring the airway remains open.

2. **Compression Technique:** When performing chest compressions on an infant, use two fingers in the center of the chest, just below the nipple line. Compress the chest to a depth of about 1.5 inches at a rate of 100–120 compressions per minute.

3. **Rescue Breaths:** For infants, it's important to cover both the nose and mouth with your mouth when providing rescue breaths. Deliver gentle breaths over one second, watching for a visible chest rise.

4. **Use of AED:** If an Automated External Defibrillator (AED) is available, use pediatric pads or a pediatric dose attenuator. Follow the manufacturer's instructions for proper placement and use.

BLS for Children

Children between the ages of one and puberty requires a slightly different approach to BLS compared to infants and adults. Here are some special considerations for performing BLS on children:

1. **Compression Technique:** When performing chest compressions on a child, use the heel of one or two hands in the center of the chest, just below the nipple line. Compress the chest to a depth of about 2 inches at a rate of 100–120 compressions per minute.

2. **Rescue Breaths:** For children, provide rescue breaths by covering the child's mouth and nose with your mouth. Deliver breaths over one second, watching for a visible chest rise.

3. **Use of AED:** If an AED is available, use pediatric pads or a pediatric dose attenuator. Follow the manufacturer's instructions for proper placement and use.

BLS for the Elderly

Performing BLS on the elderly population requires some additional considerations due to age-related changes in the body. Here are some important points to keep in mind when performing BLS on the elderly:

1. **Compression Technique:** When performing chest compressions on the elderly, use the heel of one or two

hands in the center of the chest, just below the nipple line. Compress the chest to a depth of about 2 inches at a rate of 100–120 compressions per minute.

2. **Frailty and Bone Density:** Be mindful of the potential frailty and decreased bone density in the elderly. Apply the appropriate amount of pressure during compressions to avoid causing fractures or other injuries.

3. **Rescue Breaths:** Provide rescue breaths by covering the person's mouth with your mouth. If there are concerns about infectious diseases, consider using a barrier device such as a pocket mask.

4. **Use of AED:** If an AED is available, follow the manufacturer's instructions for proper placement and use. Be aware that some AEDs have specific settings for the elderly population.

It's important to note that these special considerations for different age groups are meant to complement the core principles of BLS. The primary goal remains the same: to provide high-quality chest compressions and effective rescue breaths to maintain circulation and oxygenation. By understanding and adapting to the unique needs of infants, children, and the elderly, you can increase the chances of a successful outcome during a cardiac arrest emergency.

Remember, practice and familiarity with BLS techniques through regular training and certification courses are crucial to ensuring confidence and competence when faced with a real-life emergency.

Chapter 4

Advanced Cardiac Life Support (ACLS)

The Role of ACLS in Cardiac Arrest Management

Advanced Cardiac Life Support (ACLS) plays a crucial role in the management of cardiac arrest. While Basic Life Support (BLS) focuses on the initial steps of resuscitation, ACLS takes over when more advanced interventions are required. In this section, we will explore the specific role of ACLS in cardiac arrest management and the techniques used to improve patient outcomes.

ACLS is designed to provide a systematic approach to treating cardiac arrest, restore blood circulation, and maintain oxygenation to vital organs. It involves a combination of advanced airway management, medication administration, and the recognition and treatment of cardiac arrhythmias.

One of the key components of ACLS is advanced airway management. This involves the insertion of an endotracheal tube or the use of supraglottic airway devices to secure the airway and ensure adequate oxygenation. By providing a clear and protected airway, ACLS helps to optimize oxygen delivery to the lungs and prevent further deterioration of the patient's condition.

In addition to airway management, ACLS also involves the administration of medications to support cardiac function and restore normal heart rhythm. Medications such as epinephrine, amiodarone, and vasopressin are commonly used during ACLS to improve the chances of successful resuscitation. These medications work by increasing the heart's pumping ability, stabilizing abnormal heart rhythms, and improving blood flow to vital organs.

Recognizing and treating cardiac arrhythmias is another critical aspect of ACLS. Cardiac arrest often results from a life-threatening arrhythmia, such as ventricular fibrillation or pulseless ventricular tachycardia. ACLS protocols provide guidelines for identifying these arrhythmias and delivering appropriate interventions, such as defibrillation or antiarrhythmic medications, to restore normal heart rhythm.

ACLS also emphasizes the importance of effective team dynamics and communication during resuscitation efforts. In a high-stress situation like cardiac arrest, clear communication and coordination among healthcare providers are essential for delivering timely and efficient care. ACLS training emphasizes the roles and responsibilities of each team member, ensuring that everyone works together seamlessly to maximize the chances of a successful outcome.

Furthermore, ACLS incorporates the use of advanced monitoring techniques to assess the patient's response to treatment. Continuous electrocardiogram (ECG) monitoring allows healthcare providers to monitor the patient's heart rhythm and make necessary adjustments to the treatment plan. Additionally, invasive monitoring, such as arterial lines and central venous catheters, may be utilized to closely monitor blood pressure, oxygen levels, and other vital parameters.

ACLS is not limited to the hospital setting; it is also applicable in pre-hospital and emergency medical service (EMS) settings. Paramedics and other trained personnel are equipped with the knowledge and skills to initiate ACLS interventions in the field, even before the patient reaches the hospital. This early intervention can significantly improve the chances of a positive outcome for patients experiencing cardiac arrest.

It is important to note that ACLS is not a standalone treatment but rather a continuation of the BLS chain of survival. BLS interventions, such as high-quality chest compressions and rescue breaths, must be initiated promptly to provide the foundation for successful ACLS interventions. BLS and ACLS work hand in hand to increase the likelihood of survival and minimize the risk of long-term complications.

ACLS plays a vital role in the management of cardiac arrest by providing advanced interventions beyond the scope of BLS. It involves advanced airway management, medication administration, recognition and treatment of cardiac arrhythmias, effective team dynamics, and continuous monitoring. By incorporating these elements into the resuscitation process, ACLS aims to improve patient outcomes and increase the chances of survival.

Performing Advanced Airway Management

In the previous section, we discussed the importance of advanced cardiac life support (ACLS) in managing cardiac arrest. Now, let's delve into the crucial aspect of performing advanced airway management during ACLS. When a person experiences cardiac arrest, their breathing may become compromised or cease altogether. In such cases, it is essential to establish and maintain an open airway to ensure adequate oxygenation and ventilation. This section will guide you through the techniques and considerations involved in advanced airway management.

The Importance of Airway Management

Effective airway management is vital in ACLS because it ensures the delivery of oxygen to the lungs and the removal of carbon dioxide. By establishing an open airway, you can facilitate the exchange of gases necessary for the body's vital functions. Additionally, maintaining a patent airway allows for the administration of rescue breaths and the use of advanced airway devices, such as endotracheal tubes or supraglottic airways.

Assessing the Airway

Before initiating advanced airway management, it is crucial to assess the patient's airway. The primary goal is to determine if the airway is open or obstructed. Look for signs of airway obstruction, such as snoring, gurgling, or the absence of breath sounds. If the patient is unresponsive and not breathing or only gasping, assume that the airway is compromised and take immediate action.

Basic Airway Maneuvers

In some cases, basic airway maneuvers may be sufficient to open the airway and restore breathing. The most commonly used maneuvers are the head tilt-chin lift and the jaw thrust.

1. **Head Tilt-Chin Lift:** Place one hand on the patient's forehead and gently tilt their head back while lifting the chin with your other hand. This maneuver helps to align the airway and open the passage for air to flow.
2. **Jaw Thrust:** If there is a suspected neck injury, use the jaw thrust maneuver instead. Place your fingers behind the angles of the patient's lower jaw and lift it forward, displacing the jaw without tilting the head. This technique helps to maintain the alignment of the

airway without potentially exacerbating any neck injuries.

Advanced Airway Techniques

In some cases, basic airway maneuvers may not be sufficient, especially if the patient is not breathing adequately or if advanced airway management is required. Advanced airway techniques involve the use of specialized devices to secure the airway and provide better control over ventilation. Two commonly used advanced airway techniques are endotracheal intubation and the use of supraglottic airways.

1. **Endotracheal Intubation:** Endotracheal intubation involves the insertion of an endotracheal tube through the mouth or nose into the trachea. This technique provides a secure airway and allows for precise control over ventilation. However, it requires specialized training and expertise to perform correctly. It is essential to confirm the tube's placement using methods such as auscultation, capnography, or chest rise.

2. **Supraglottic Airways:** Supraglottic airways, such as the laryngeal mask airway (LMA) or the King LT airway, are alternative devices used for advanced airway management. These devices are inserted into the oropharynx and provide a seal around the larynx, allowing for ventilation. Supraglottic airways are

easier to insert than endotracheal tubes and can be used by healthcare providers with varying levels of expertise.

Considerations for Airway Management

When performing advanced airway management, several considerations should be kept in mind to ensure patient safety and optimize outcomes.

1. **Continuous Monitoring:** Once an advanced airway is in place, continuous monitoring of the patient's oxygenation, ventilation, and end-tidal carbon dioxide (ETCO2) levels is crucial. This monitoring helps to assess the effectiveness of ventilation and detect any complications promptly.

2. **Securing the Airway:** After intubation or placement of a supraglottic airway, it is essential to secure the device properly to prevent accidental dislodgement. Use appropriate methods, such as securing the endotracheal tube with tape or using the provided fixation device for supraglottic airways.

3. **Avoiding Hyperventilation:** During ventilation, it is important to avoid hyperventilation, as it can lead to complications such as decreased cardiac output and increased intrathoracic pressure. Follow the recommended ventilation rates and tidal volumes to ensure adequate oxygenation without causing harm.

4. **Considering Alternative Techniques:** In some situations, advanced airway management may not be feasible or appropriate. For example, in cases of severe facial trauma or airway obstruction, alternative techniques like needle cricothyroidotomy or surgical cricothyroidotomy may be necessary. These techniques should only be performed by healthcare providers with the appropriate training and expertise.

Performing advanced airway management is a critical component of ACLS. By assessing the airway, using basic maneuvers, and employing advanced techniques such as endotracheal intubation or supraglottic airways, you can establish and maintain a patent airway to ensure adequate oxygenation and ventilation.

Continuous monitoring, proper securing of the airway, and avoiding hyperventilation are essential considerations during advanced airway management. Remember to consider alternative techniques when necessary and always prioritize patient safety and optimal outcomes.

Administering Medications during ACLS

Administering medications is a crucial aspect of advanced cardiac life support (ACLS) during a cardiac arrest. These medications are used to restore and maintain the heart's rhythm, improve blood flow, and increase the chances of a successful resuscitation. In this section, we will explore the different medications used in ACLS and their administration.

Medications Used in ACLS

There are several medications commonly used in ACLS, each serving a specific purpose in the resuscitation process. Let's take a closer look at some of these medications:

1. **Epinephrine:** Epinephrine is a medication that plays a vital role in ACLS. It is a potent vasoconstrictor, which means it narrows the blood vessels, increasing blood pressure and improving blood flow to the heart and brain. Epinephrine is administered intravenously during cardiac arrest to help restore a stable heart rhythm.

2. **Amiodarone:** Amiodarone is an antiarrhythmic medication used to treat life-threatening ventricular arrhythmias, such as ventricular fibrillation or pulseless ventricular tachycardia. It works by stabilizing the heart's electrical activity and restoring a normal rhythm. Amiodarone is typically administered intravenously during ACLS.

3. **Lidocaine:** Lidocaine is another antiarrhythmic medication used in ACLS. It is primarily used to treat ventricular arrhythmias that are resistant to other treatments. Lidocaine works by blocking abnormal electrical signals in the heart, helping to restore a

normal rhythm. It is administered intravenously during cardiac arrest.

4. **Atropine:** Atropine is a medication used to treat symptomatic bradycardia, a condition characterized by a slow heart rate. It works by blocking certain nerve impulses and increasing the heart rate. Atropine is typically administered intravenously during ACLS to help restore a normal heart rhythm.

5. **Adenosine:** Adenosine is a medication used to treat supraventricular tachycardia (SVT), a rapid heart rhythm originating above the ventricles. It works by slowing down the electrical conduction in the heart, allowing the normal rhythm to resume. Adenosine is administered rapidly through an intravenous bolus during ACLS.

6. **Magnesium sulfate:** Magnesium sulfate is a medication used to treat certain types of arrhythmias, such as torsades de pointes, which is a specific form of ventricular tachycardia. It works by stabilizing the electrical activity of the heart. Magnesium sulfate is typically administered intravenously during ACLS.

Medication Administration

Administering medications during ACLS requires proper training and understanding of the specific protocols. Here are some important considerations for medication administration:

1. **Dosage and Route:** Each medication has a specific dosage and route of administration. It is crucial to follow the recommended dosages and routes to ensure the medication's effectiveness and minimize the risk of adverse effects. Intravenous administration is the most common route during ACLS, as it allows for rapid absorption and immediate effect.

2. **Compatibility:** Some medications may interact with each other, leading to adverse effects or reduced efficacy. It is essential to check for compatibility before administering multiple medications simultaneously. Your ACLS training will provide guidance on which medications can be safely administered together.

3. **Monitoring:** After administering a medication, it is crucial to closely monitor the patient's response. Monitoring includes assessing vital signs, electrocardiogram (ECG) readings, and overall clinical status. This helps determine the effectiveness of the medication and guides further interventions if needed.

4. **Adverse Effects:** Like any medication, ACLS medications can have potential adverse effects. It is important to be aware of these effects and monitor the patient for any signs of complications. Common adverse effects may include allergic reactions, changes in blood pressure, or arrhythmias.

5. **Documentation:** Accurate documentation of medication administration is essential for continuity of care and legal purposes. Document the medication name, dosage, route, time of administration, and the patient's response. This information helps healthcare providers track the patient's progress and make informed decisions.

Special Considerations

In certain situations, special considerations must be taken into account when administering medications during ACLS. Here are a few examples:

1. **Pregnancy:** When managing cardiac arrest in pregnant patients, the safety of both the mother and the fetus must be considered. Some medications, such as epinephrine and amiodarone, are generally considered safe for use during pregnancy. However, the dosage and administration may need to be adjusted based on the gestational age and the specific circumstances.

2. **Elderly Population:** Older adults may have different medication requirements and may be more susceptible to adverse effects. Careful consideration should be given to the choice of medications and their dosages in the elderly population. Close monitoring is essential to ensure the medications are well-tolerated and effective.

3. **Drug Interactions:** Patients may be taking other medications that can interact with ACLS medications. It is crucial to review the patient's medication history and consider potential drug interactions before administering ACLS medications. Consultation with a pharmacist or healthcare provider may be necessary in complex cases.

4. **Allergies and Sensitivities:** Some patients may have known allergies or sensitivities to specific medications. It is important to inquire about any known allergies before administering medications. If an allergic reaction occurs, appropriate interventions, such as administering epinephrine or antihistamines, should be initiated promptly.

Remember, medication administration during ACLS should only be performed by trained healthcare professionals who are authorized to do so. The proper use of medications, along with other ACLS interventions, can significantly improve the chances of successful resuscitation and save lives.

In the next section, we will explore the recognition and treatment of cardiac arrhythmias during ACLS.

Recognizing and Treating Cardiac Arrhythmias

Cardiac arrhythmias are abnormal heart rhythms that can occur during a cardiac arrest or as a result of various underlying medical conditions. These irregular heart rhythms can be life-threatening and require immediate recognition and treatment during cardiopulmonary resuscitation (CPR). In this section, we will explore the different types of cardiac arrhythmias, their causes, and the appropriate interventions to manage them effectively.

Types of Cardiac Arrhythmias

Several types of cardiac arrhythmias can occur during a cardiac arrest. Healthcare providers must be able to recognize these arrhythmias and provide the appropriate treatment. Here are some of the most common types:

1. **Ventricular Fibrillation (VF):** VF is a chaotic and disorganized rhythm that prevents the heart from effectively pumping blood. It is a leading cause of sudden cardiac arrest and requires immediate defibrillation.

2. **Ventricular Tachycardia (VT):** VT is a rapid heart rhythm originating from the ventricles. It can be sustained or non-sustained and may deteriorate into VF if left untreated.

3. **Asystole:** Asystole, also known as "flatline," is the absence of any electrical activity in the heart. It is a life-threatening condition that requires immediate intervention.

4. **Pulseless Electrical Activity (PEA):** PEA is characterized by the presence of electrical activity in the heart without a detectable pulse. It is essential to identify and treat the underlying cause of PEA to restore a perfusing rhythm.

Causes of Cardiac Arrhythmias

Cardiac arrhythmias can occur due to various factors, including underlying heart conditions, electrolyte imbalances, drug toxicity, and other medical emergencies. Understanding the potential causes can help healthcare providers identify and address the underlying issue. Here are some common causes of cardiac arrhythmias:

1. **Ischemic Heart Disease:** Coronary artery disease and myocardial infarction can disrupt the heart's electrical system, leading to arrhythmias.
2. **Electrolyte Imbalances:** Abnormal levels of potassium, calcium, or magnesium in the blood can affect the heart's electrical conduction system and trigger arrhythmias.
3. **Drug Toxicity:** Certain medications, such as antiarrhythmics, beta-blockers, and digitalis, can cause arrhythmias as a side effect or due to an overdose.
4. **Cardiomyopathy:** Conditions that weaken the heart muscle, such as dilated cardiomyopathy or

hypertrophic cardiomyopathy, can disrupt the heart's electrical signals.

5. **Hypoxia:** Lack of oxygen supply to the heart, often seen in cardiac arrest or respiratory failure, can lead to arrhythmias.

Recognizing Cardiac Arrhythmias

Recognizing cardiac arrhythmias is crucial for providing appropriate treatment during CPR. Healthcare providers should be able to identify abnormal heart rhythms through various means, including clinical signs, symptoms, and electrocardiogram (ECG) monitoring. Here are some key points to consider when recognizing cardiac arrhythmias:

1. **Assessing the Patient:** Evaluate the patient's level of consciousness, pulse, and breathing. Look for signs of inadequate perfusion, such as pale skin, cool extremities, and altered mental status.

2. **Monitoring the ECG:** Continuous ECG monitoring provides real-time information about the heart's electrical activity. Look for irregularities in the rhythm, abnormal QRS complexes, and the absence of P waves.

3. **Analyzing the Rhythm:** Determine the heart rhythm by assessing the intervals between QRS complexes, the presence or absence of P waves, and the overall pattern on the ECG.

4. **Identifying Life-Threatening Arrhythmias:** Focus on identifying VF, VT, asystole, and PEA, as these require immediate intervention.

Treating Cardiac Arrhythmias

The treatment of cardiac arrhythmias during CPR depends on the specific rhythm and the patient's condition. Prompt intervention is essential to restore a perfusing rhythm and improve the chances of survival. Here are some key interventions for treating cardiac arrhythmias:

1. **Defibrillation:** For VF and pulseless VT, immediate defibrillation is the primary treatment. Deliver an electric shock using an automated external defibrillator (AED) or manual defibrillator to restore a normal rhythm.
2. **CPR with High-Quality Chest Compressions:** In the absence of a shockable rhythm, perform high-quality chest compressions to maintain blood flow to vital organs. CPR should be continued until a defibrillator is available or advanced medical support arrives.
3. **Medications:** In certain cases, medications may be administered to manage specific arrhythmias. These medications include antiarrhythmics, vasopressors, and electrolyte replacements.
4. **Advanced Airway Management:** Consider advanced airway interventions, such as endotracheal intubation

or supraglottic airway placement, to optimize oxygenation and ventilation during CPR.

5. **Addressing Underlying Causes:** Identify and address the underlying cause of the arrhythmia, such as myocardial infarction, electrolyte imbalances, or drug toxicity.

Remember, the treatment of cardiac arrhythmias during CPR requires a systematic approach and the ability to adapt to the patient's condition. Regular training and practice are essential to developing the necessary skills and confidence to manage these life-threatening situations effectively.

Chapter 5

Pediatric Cardiopulmonary Resuscitation

Differences and Similarities between Adult and Pediatric CPR

When it comes to performing cardiopulmonary resuscitation (CPR), there are some key differences and similarities between adult and pediatric cases. While the overall goal remains the same—to restore blood circulation and oxygenation to the body—some specific techniques and considerations need to be taken into account when performing CPR on infants and children.

Differences in Anatomy and Physiology

One of the primary differences between adult and pediatric CPR lies in the anatomy and physiology of the patients. Infants and children have smaller and more delicate bodies, which means that the techniques used in adult CPR may not be suitable for them. Here are some key differences to keep in mind:

1. Chest Compressions

In adult CPR, chest compressions are performed by placing the heel of one hand on the center of the chest and interlocking the fingers. However, in pediatric CPR, the rescuer should use two or three fingers instead of the full hand. The depth of compressions also differs, with the recommended depth being about one-third to one-half the depth of the chest for infants and about one-third the depth for children.

2. Rescue Breaths

When it comes to rescue breaths, the technique varies between adults and children. In adult CPR, the rescuer provides two breaths after every 30 compressions. However, in pediatric CPR, the ratio changes to 30 compressions followed by two breaths for infants and children. It's important to note that the volume of breath should be smaller for infants and children compared to adults.

3. AED Use

Automated External Defibrillators (AEDs) are commonly used in CPR to deliver an electric shock to the heart in cases of cardiac arrest. While AEDs can be used on both adults and children, there are specific pediatric pads or settings available for children under the age of eight. These pads or settings deliver a lower energy shock suitable for their smaller bodies.

Differences in Etiology and Causes of Cardiac Arrest

The causes of cardiac arrest in adults and children can vary significantly. In adults, cardiac arrest is often the result of underlying heart conditions, such as coronary artery disease or arrhythmias. On the other hand, in children, cardiac arrest is more commonly caused by respiratory issues such as choking, drowning, or severe infections.

Differences in Response and Recognition

Recognizing cardiac arrest in adults and children can also differ. In adults, the signs of cardiac arrest are often more apparent, with the person suddenly collapsing and losing consciousness. However, in infants and children, the signs may be subtler, such as a change in skin color, difficulty breathing, or a weak pulse. Rescuers must be vigilant and aware of these differences to ensure prompt recognition and initiation of CPR.

Similarities in Basic CPR Steps

While there are notable differences, the basic steps of CPR remain the same for both adults and children. These steps include:

1. **Assessing the situation and ensuring safety:** Before initiating CPR, it's important to ensure that the scene is safe for both the rescuer and the patient.
2. **Activating emergency medical services (EMS):** Calling for professional help is crucial in any CPR

situation. The sooner professional medical assistance arrives, the better the chances of a positive outcome.

3. **Performing chest compressions:** The primary goal of CPR is to restore blood circulation. This is achieved through high-quality chest compressions, regardless of the age of the patient.

4. **Providing rescue breaths:** In addition to chest compressions, rescue breaths are given to provide oxygen to the patient's lungs and body.

5. **Using an AED if available:** If an AED is accessible, it should be used as soon as possible to deliver a shock if necessary.

Performing CPR on infants and children requires specific techniques and considerations due to their unique anatomy, physiology, and causes of cardiac arrest. While there are differences between adult and pediatric CPR, the overall goal remains the same; to restore blood circulation and oxygenation to the body. By understanding these differences and similarities, rescuers can be better prepared to provide effective CPR and potentially save lives.

Performing CPR on Infants and Children

Performing cardiopulmonary resuscitation (CPR) on infants and children requires a slightly different approach compared to adults. Their smaller size and unique physiology necessitate specific techniques to ensure effective resuscitation. In this section, we will explore the key considerations and steps involved in performing CPR on infants and children.

Understanding the Differences

Before diving into the specifics of CPR for infants and children, it's important to understand the key differences between adult and pediatric resuscitation. Infants are defined as children under the age of one, while children refer to those between the ages of one and puberty.

One significant difference is the cause of cardiac arrest. In adults, cardiac arrest is often due to a heart-related issue, such as a heart attack. However, in infants and children, cardiac arrest is commonly caused by respiratory failure or shock. Therefore, the focus of pediatric CPR is on addressing these underlying causes while providing effective chest compressions and rescue breaths.

Step-by-Step Guide to Pediatric CPR

Performing CPR on infants and children follows a similar sequence of steps as adult CPR, with a few modifications. Let's walk through the process:

1. **Assess the situation and ensure safety:** Before initiating CPR, assess the scene for any potential dangers. Ensure that both you and the child are in a safe environment.

2. **Check for responsiveness:** Tap the child's shoulder and shout their name to check for responsiveness. If there is no response, gently shake their shoulders.

3. **Activate emergency medical services (EMS):** If the child is unresponsive, immediately activate EMS or ask someone nearby to do so. Time is of the essence in pediatric cardiac arrest cases.

4. **Open the airway:** Place the child on their back on a firm surface. Tilt their head back slightly to open the airway. Remember, in infants, to avoid hyperextending the neck.

5. **Check for breathing:** Look, listen, and feel for any signs of breathing for no more than ten seconds. If the child is not breathing or is only gasping, proceed to the next step.

6. **Perform chest compressions:** For infants, use two fingers to deliver chest compressions. Place your fingers on the lower half of the breastbone and compress the chest about 1.5 inches deep at a rate of 100–120 compressions per minute. For children, use the heel of one or two hands and compress the chest about 2 inches deep.

7. **Provide rescue breaths:** After 30 compressions, give two rescue breaths. For infants, cover both the nose and mouth with your mouth and deliver gentle breaths.

For children, cover only the mouth and provide breaths that make the chest rise visibly.

8. **Continue cycles of compressions and breaths:** Repeat the cycle of 30 compressions followed by two breaths until help arrives or the child shows signs of recovery.

Special Considerations for Infants

When performing CPR on infants, there are a few additional considerations to keep in mind:

1. **Head positioning:** As mentioned earlier, avoid hyperextending the neck. Instead, maintain a neutral position to ensure a patent airway.
2. **Compression technique:** Use the two-finger technique for chest compressions in infants. Place your index and middle fingers on the lower half of the breastbone, just below the nipple line.
3. **Rescue breaths:** Cover both the infant's nose and mouth with your mouth to provide rescue breaths. Ensure a good seal and deliver gentle breaths.

Special Considerations for Children

When performing CPR on children, consider the following:

1. **Compression technique:** Use the heel of one or two hands for chest compressions. Place your hands on the

lower half of the breastbone, just above the xiphoid process.

2. **Rescue breaths:** Cover only the child's mouth with your mouth to provide rescue breaths. Ensure a good seal and deliver breaths that visibly make the chest rise.

A Word on AED Use

Automated External Defibrillators (AEDs) can be used for infants and children in cardiac arrest. However, it's important to use pediatric-specific pads or a pediatric attenuator when available. These modifications ensure that the energy delivered by the AED is appropriate for the child's size.

Performing CPR on infants and children requires a slightly different approach compared to adults. Understanding the key differences and following the appropriate steps is crucial for providing effective resuscitation. By being prepared and knowledgeable, you can make a significant difference in saving the lives of infants and children in cardiac arrest.

Managing Pediatric Cardiac Arrest in Special Circumstances

When it comes to managing pediatric cardiac arrest, certain special circumstances require specific considerations and techniques. Children have unique physiological and anatomical differences compared to adults, which means that their resuscitation needs may vary. In this section, we will explore some of these special circumstances and discuss how to effectively manage pediatric cardiac arrest in these situations.

Newborn Resuscitation

Newborn resuscitation is a critical aspect of pediatric cardiac arrest management. It is essential to be prepared for any complications that may arise during childbirth or in the immediate postnatal period. The key steps in newborn resuscitation include:

1. **Clearing the airway:** Ensure that the newborn's airway is clear of any obstructions, such as mucus or amniotic fluid. Gently suction the mouth and nose, if necessary.

2. **Providing positive pressure ventilation:** If the newborn is not breathing or has inadequate respiratory effort, provide positive pressure ventilation using a bag-mask device or a specialized neonatal resuscitation device. Use gentle and controlled breaths to avoid causing harm.

3. **Performing chest compressions:** If the newborn's heart rate remains below the desired range despite adequate ventilation, initiate chest compressions. Use two fingers to compress the chest at a rate of 120

compressions per minute, with a depth of approximately one-third the depth of the chest.

4. **Administering medications:** In certain cases, medications such as epinephrine may be required to support the newborn's circulation. Follow the appropriate dosages and administration guidelines.

Pediatric Cardiac Arrest in the Hospital Setting

Pediatric cardiac arrest can occur in various hospital settings, including emergency departments, intensive care units, and operating rooms. In these situations, it is crucial to have a well-coordinated response to maximize the chances of a successful resuscitation. Some considerations for managing pediatric cardiac arrest in the hospital setting include:

1. **Rapid response teams:** Many hospitals have rapid response teams specifically trained to respond to pediatric emergencies. These teams consist of healthcare professionals with expertise in pediatric resuscitation. Activating the rapid response team promptly can significantly improve the outcome for the child.

2. **Effective communication:** Clear and concise communication among the healthcare team is vital during a pediatric cardiac arrest. Assign specific roles to team members, ensure everyone understands their

responsibilities, and use closed-loop communication to relay critical information.

3. **Utilizing pediatric-specific equipment:** Hospitals should have pediatric-specific equipment readily available, including appropriately sized airway devices, defibrillator pads, and medication dosages. Ensure that the equipment is regularly checked, maintained, and easily accessible in case of an emergency.

4. **Adapting to the child's size and weight:** When performing chest compressions, it is essential to adjust the technique based on the child's size and weight. Use two hands for infants and smaller children, and transition to one hand for older children. The depth and rate of compression should also be adjusted accordingly.

Pediatric Cardiac Arrest in the Pre-hospital Setting

Pediatric cardiac arrest can also occur outside of the hospital, requiring immediate attention and intervention. In the pre-hospital setting, emergency medical services (EMS) play a crucial role in managing pediatric cardiac arrest. Here are some considerations for managing pediatric cardiac arrest in the pre-hospital setting:

1. **Early activation of EMS:** As soon as a pediatric cardiac arrest is identified, activate EMS immediately.

Time is of the essence, and early intervention can significantly improve the child's chances of survival.

2. **CPR initiation by bystanders:** If there are bystanders present at the scene, encourage them to initiate CPR promptly. Bystander CPR has been shown to improve outcomes in pediatric cardiac arrest cases. Provide clear and concise instructions on how to perform CPR until EMS arrives.

3. **Utilizing pediatric-specific AEDs:** Automated External Defibrillators (AEDs) are essential in managing cardiac arrest. In the case of pediatric cardiac arrest, it is crucial to use pediatric-specific AED pads or equipment that can deliver appropriate energy levels for children.

4. **Transportation considerations:** When transporting a child in cardiac arrest, it is important to ensure continuous CPR and appropriate ventilation. Secure the child safely in the ambulance and continue resuscitation efforts during transportation to the hospital.

Pediatric Cardiac Arrest in Special Populations

Certain populations of children may have unique considerations when it comes to managing cardiac arrest. These populations include children with underlying medical conditions, those with special healthcare needs, or those who are victims of trauma or abuse. Some key points to consider in managing pediatric cardiac arrest in special populations include:

1. **Individualized care:** Children with underlying medical conditions or special healthcare needs may require individualized care during resuscitation. Consider their specific medical history, any known allergies, and any potential complications that may arise due to their condition.

2. **Trauma-related cardiac arrest:** In cases of trauma-related cardiac arrest, it is crucial to address any life-threatening injuries while simultaneously providing CPR. Control bleeding, immobilize the spine if necessary, and ensure a clear airway.

3. **Child abuse and neglect:** Pediatric cardiac arrest resulting from abuse or neglect requires a multidisciplinary approach involving healthcare professionals, social workers, and law enforcement. Document any suspicious findings and report them to the appropriate authorities.

Remember, managing pediatric cardiac arrest in special circumstances requires a combination of knowledge, skill, and adaptability. Stay calm, follow the appropriate protocols, and work as a team to provide the best possible care for the child in need.

Preventing Pediatric Cardiac Arrest

Preventing pediatric cardiac arrest is a crucial aspect of ensuring the well-being and safety of children. While it may not always be possible to prevent cardiac arrest entirely, several measures can significantly reduce the risk and increase the chances of a positive outcome in case of an emergency. In this section, we will explore various strategies and practices that can help prevent pediatric cardiac arrest.

1. Promoting a Healthy Lifestyle

One of the most effective ways to prevent pediatric cardiac arrest is by promoting a healthy lifestyle for children. This includes encouraging regular physical activity, maintaining a balanced diet, and ensuring adequate sleep. By engaging in regular exercise, children can strengthen their cardiovascular system, reducing the risk of cardiac events. Additionally, a healthy diet rich in fruits, vegetables, and whole grains provides essential nutrients that support heart health.

2. Childproofing the Environment

Accidents and injuries are common causes of pediatric cardiac arrest. Childproofing the environment is essential to minimize the risk of accidents and create a safe space for children. This involves securing furniture and appliances to prevent tipping, installing safety gates and window guards, and keeping hazardous substances out of reach. By creating a child-friendly environment, the chances of accidents leading to cardiac arrest can be significantly reduced.

3. Supervision and Education

Supervision and education play a vital role in preventing pediatric cardiac arrest. Parents, caregivers, and educators must be vigilant and provide constant supervision, especially around water bodies, during playtime, and in potentially dangerous situations. Educating children about potential risks and teaching them basic safety measures, such as wearing helmets while cycling or using seat belts in vehicles, can empower them to make safer choices.

4. Immunizations and Regular Check-ups

Immunizations and regular check-ups are essential components of preventive healthcare for children. Vaccinations protect against various diseases, some of which can lead to cardiac complications. By ensuring that children receive their recommended immunizations, the risk of cardiac arrest due to preventable diseases can be significantly reduced. Regular check-ups with healthcare professionals also allow for the early detection and management of any underlying conditions that may increase the risk of cardiac events.

5. CPR and First Aid Training

Equipping parents, caregivers, and educators with CPR and first aid training is crucial to preventing pediatric cardiac arrest. By learning these life-saving techniques, individuals can respond promptly and effectively in case of an emergency. CPR training teaches the proper techniques for performing chest compressions and rescue breaths, which can help maintain blood circulation and oxygenation until medical professionals arrive. First aid training provides knowledge on how to manage injuries and stabilize a child's condition until further medical assistance is available.

6. Water Safety

Drowning is a leading cause of pediatric cardiac arrest, particularly in young children. Implementing water safety measures is essential to preventing such incidents. This includes constant supervision around water bodies, ensuring the presence of barriers such as fences around pools, and teaching children how to swim at an appropriate age. Additionally, it is crucial to educate children about the dangers of water and the importance of following safety rules, such as not swimming alone or diving into unknown waters.

7. Safe Sleep Practices

Sudden Infant Death Syndrome (SIDS) is a significant concern for infants and can lead to cardiac arrest. Implementing safe sleep practices can help reduce the risk of SIDS. This includes placing infants on their backs to sleep, using a firm mattress and a fitted sheet in the crib, avoiding loose bedding and soft objects, and keeping the sleeping area free from hazards such as cords or toys. By following these guidelines, the risk of SIDS and subsequent cardiac arrest can be minimized.

8. Managing Underlying Medical Conditions

Some children may have underlying medical conditions that increase their risk of cardiac arrest. It is crucial to manage these conditions effectively to prevent cardiac events. This may involve regular medical follow-ups, adherence to prescribed medications, and lifestyle modifications as recommended by healthcare professionals. By effectively managing underlying medical conditions, the risk of cardiac arrest can be significantly reduced.

9. Emergency Preparedness

Being prepared for emergencies is essential to preventing pediatric cardiac arrest. This includes having a well-stocked first aid kit readily available, knowing the location of the nearest emergency medical services, and having emergency contact numbers easily accessible. It is also important to have a plan in place for emergencies, including knowing how to perform CPR and when to activate emergency medical services. By being prepared, individuals can respond quickly and effectively in critical situations.

10. Creating a Supportive Environment

Creating a supportive environment for children is crucial to preventing pediatric cardiac arrest. This involves fostering open communication, providing emotional support, and promoting mental well-being. By addressing emotional and psychological needs, children are less likely to engage in risky behaviors or experience excessive stress, which can contribute to cardiac events. Creating a supportive environment also involves promoting positive relationships and healthy coping mechanisms.

Promoting a healthy lifestyle, childproofing the environment, providing supervision and education, ensuring regular check-ups and immunizations, offering CPR and first aid training, implementing water safety measures, following safe sleep practices, managing underlying medical conditions, being prepared for emergencies, and creating a supportive environment can significantly reduce the risk of pediatric cardiac arrest. Parents, caregivers, educators, and healthcare professionals must work together to implement these preventive measures and ensure the well-being and safety of children.

Chapter 6

Special Situations and Considerations

CPR in Pregnancy and Childbirth

Pregnancy and childbirth are beautiful and miraculous events, but they can also come with unexpected complications. In some cases, a pregnant woman may experience a cardiac arrest or other life-threatening emergencies during pregnancy or labor. As a healthcare provider or a bystander, it is crucial to be prepared and knowledgeable about performing CPR in these unique situations. In this section, we will explore the specific considerations and techniques for CPR in pregnancy and childbirth.

Understanding the Physiology

Before we delve into the specifics of CPR in pregnancy and childbirth, it is essential to understand the physiological changes that occur in a pregnant woman's body. During pregnancy, the woman's blood volume increases, and her heart rate and cardiac output also rise. Additionally, the growing uterus can compress the inferior vena cava, reducing blood return to the heart. These changes can affect the effectiveness of CPR techniques and require modifications to ensure the safety of both the mother and the baby.

Assessing the Situation

When encountering a pregnant woman in cardiac arrest or distress, it is crucial to assess the situation promptly. Ensure that the scene is safe for both you and the patient. If possible, activate the emergency medical services (EMS) immediately to ensure professional help arrives as soon as possible. Remember, time is of the essence in these situations.

Modifying CPR Techniques

Performing CPR on a pregnant woman requires some modifications to accommodate the physiological changes and protect the developing fetus. Here are some key considerations:

1. **Positioning:** Position the pregnant woman on her left side to relieve pressure on the inferior vena cava and improve blood flow to the heart. This position helps maintain blood supply to the placenta and the baby.
2. **Chest Compressions:** Place your hands on the lower half of the woman's sternum, just like in standard CPR. However, you may need to compress the chest slightly higher than usual to account for the upward displacement of the diaphragm caused by the growing uterus.

3. **Rescue Breaths:** Provide rescue breaths with caution, as the pressure exerted during ventilation can potentially harm the fetus. Use a barrier device or a face mask with an oxygen reservoir to minimize direct contact and reduce the risk of infection.

4. **Compression-to-Ventilation Ratio:** The standard compression-to-ventilation ratio of 30:2 still applies in CPR for pregnant women. However, if there are concerns about the fetus's well-being, consider increasing the number of compressions per minute while maintaining adequate ventilation.

Special Considerations for Childbirth

Childbirth is a unique situation that requires additional considerations when performing CPR. Here are some important points to keep in mind:

1. **Delivery:** If the pregnant woman is in labor and the baby's head is visible, prepare for delivery. Support the baby's head and neck during delivery to prevent any potential injuries. Once the baby is delivered, assess the condition and provide immediate care if needed.

2. **Umbilical Cord:** If the umbilical cord is wrapped around the baby's neck, gently slip it over the baby's head to relieve any potential obstruction to breathing. Be cautious not to pull or tug on the cord forcefully.

3. **Neonatal Resuscitation:** If the baby is not breathing or is in distress after delivery, initiate neonatal resuscitation following the appropriate guidelines. This may involve providing chest compressions, clearing the airway, and providing rescue breaths to the newborn.

Communicating with the Mother

During these critical moments, it is essential to communicate with the mother or any available family members. Explain the situation clearly and provide reassurance. Keep them informed about the steps you are taking and the progress of the resuscitation efforts. Compassion and empathy can go a long way in these emotionally charged situations.

Legal and Ethical Considerations

Performing CPR in pregnancy and childbirth situations raises unique legal and ethical considerations. It is crucial to be aware of local laws and regulations regarding the provision of emergency care to pregnant women and newborns. Additionally, respecting the mother's autonomy and involving her in decision-making, if possible, is essential.

Training and Preparation

Given the complexity and unique challenges of performing CPR during pregnancy and childbirth, healthcare providers need to receive specialized training in this area. Organizations such as the American Heart Association offer courses that specifically address CPR during pregnancy and childbirth. By staying updated and prepared, you can enhance your ability to provide effective and safe care in these critical situations.

Remember, every second counts when it comes to saving lives. Being knowledgeable and confident in performing CPR during pregnancy and childbirth can make a significant difference in the outcomes for both the mother and the baby.

CPR in Drowning and Near-Drowning Incidents

Drowning and near-drowning incidents are terrifying and can happen in an instant. Whether it occurs in a pool, lake, or bathtub, the outcome can be devastating if immediate action is not taken. In these situations, performing cardiopulmonary resuscitation (CPR) can be the difference between life and death.

Understanding Drowning and Near-Drowning

Drowning occurs when a person's airway is blocked, preventing them from breathing. This can happen due to submersion in water or other fluids, leading to a lack of oxygen supply to the brain and other vital organs. Near drowning refers to a situation where a person has been rescued from drowning but still requires medical intervention.

Assessing the Situation

When encountering a drowning or near-drowning incident, it is crucial to assess the situation quickly and ensure your safety before providing assistance. If the person is still in the water, it is essential to remove them from the water as soon as possible, taking care to support their head and neck to avoid any potential spinal injuries.

Activating Emergency Medical Services (EMS)

Once the person is out of the water, immediately activate emergency medical services (EMS) by calling the local emergency number. Time is of the essence in these situations, and professional medical help is necessary to provide advanced care.

Performing CPR

1. **Check for responsiveness:** Before starting CPR, check if the person is responsive by tapping their shoulder and asking if they are okay. If there is no response, proceed to the next step.

2. **Open the airway:** Tilt the person's head back gently and lift their chin to open the airway. Look, listen, and feel for any signs of breathing for no more than 10 seconds. If there is no breathing or only gasping, it is crucial to start CPR immediately.

3. **Perform chest compressions:** Place the heel of one hand on the center of the person's chest, slightly above

the lower half of the breastbone. Place your other hand on top of the first hand and interlock your fingers. Keep your elbows straight and position your shoulders directly above your hands. Push hard and fast, aiming for a compression depth of at least 2 inches. Perform compressions at a rate of 100–120 compressions per minute, allowing the chest to fully recoil between compressions.

4. **Provide rescue breaths:** After 30 compressions, give two rescue breaths. Ensure the person's airway is open, pinch their nose shut, and make a complete seal over their mouth with your mouth. Deliver each breath over one second, watching for the chest to rise. If the chest does not rise, reposition the head and try again. Continue cycles of 30 compressions and two breaths until help arrives or the person shows signs of life.

Using an Automated External Defibrillator (AED)

If an automated external defibrillator (AED) is available, it should be used as soon as possible. AEDs are portable devices that can analyze the heart's rhythm and deliver an electric shock if necessary.

Follow the instructions provided with the AED and attach the pads to the person's bare chest as directed. Ensure that no one is touching the person while the AED is analyzing or delivering a shock.

Special Considerations

When performing CPR in drowning and near-drowning incidents, there are a few special considerations to keep in mind:

1. **Water removal:** If the person has water in their airway, it is essential to clear it before starting CPR. Tilt the person's head to the side and allow any water to drain out. If necessary, use your fingers to sweep out any visible obstructions.

2. **Hypothermia:** In cold water incidents, the person may be hypothermic. Hypothermia can affect the success of CPR, so it is crucial to remove wet clothing and cover the person with a dry blanket or clothing if available. Focus on warming the person gradually and continuing CPR.

3. **Transportation:** If the person is in a remote location or far from medical help, it may be necessary to transport them while performing CPR. Coordinate with others to ensure a smooth transition and continue CPR during transportation.

4. **Emotional support:** Drowning and near-drowning incidents can be traumatic for everyone involved. Offer emotional support to the person's family and friends, as well as to yourself and any witnesses. Seek professional help if needed to process the emotional impact of the incident.

Remember, the steps outlined here are a general guide for performing CPR in drowning and near-drowning incidents. It is essential to stay updated with the latest CPR guidelines and receive proper training to ensure you are prepared to handle these emergencies effectively.

CPR in Traumatic Injuries

When it comes to cardiopulmonary resuscitation (CPR), most people associate it with cardiac arrest or respiratory emergencies. However, CPR is also crucial in traumatic injuries, where immediate intervention can mean the difference between life and death. In this section, we will explore the unique considerations and techniques involved in performing CPR in traumatic situations.

Understanding Traumatic Injuries

Traumatic injuries occur as a result of accidents, falls, sports-related incidents, or violence. These injuries can range from minor cuts and bruises to severe trauma, such as fractures, head injuries, or internal bleeding. In some cases, traumatic injuries can lead to cardiac arrest or respiratory failure, requiring prompt CPR to maintain blood circulation and oxygenation.

Assessing the Situation

Before initiating CPR in a traumatic injury scenario, it is crucial to assess the situation and ensure your safety. Ensure that the scene is safe and free from any ongoing danger, such as traffic or unstable structures. If necessary, call for help and activate emergency medical services (EMS) before proceeding with CPR.

Modified CPR Techniques

Performing CPR on traumatic injuries requires some modifications to the standard techniques. Here are a few key considerations:

1. Chest Compressions

When providing chest compressions, it is essential to be mindful of any potential fractures or injuries to the chest. Place your hands on the lower half of the sternum, avoiding any areas of obvious injury. If you suspect a spinal injury, use a modified technique called "hands-only CPR," where you focus solely on chest compressions without rescue breaths.

2. Airway Management

In traumatic injuries, there is a higher risk of airway obstruction due to blood, vomit, or swelling. Clearing the airway becomes a priority before initiating rescue breaths. Use the head-tilt and chin-lift maneuvers to open the airway, but be cautious not to exacerbate any potential neck or spinal injuries. If there are signs of a spinal injury, consider using the jaw thrust maneuver instead.

3. Bleeding Control

Traumatic injuries often involve significant bleeding, which can further compromise the patient's condition. If there is severe bleeding, apply direct pressure to the wound using a sterile dressing or cloth. Control the bleeding before initiating CPR, as maintaining blood circulation is crucial for the patient's survival.

Special Considerations

In certain traumatic injury scenarios, additional considerations may arise during CPR. Let's explore a few of these special situations:

1. Head and Neck Injuries

Patients with head or neck injuries require extra caution during CPR. Avoid excessive movement of the head and neck, as it can worsen spinal cord damage. If possible, stabilize the head and neck using manual immobilization techniques or cervical collars before initiating CPR.

2. Chest Trauma

In cases of severe chest trauma, such as rib fractures or punctured lungs, the risk of complications during CPR increases. Be mindful of any unusual chest movements or sounds, which may indicate underlying injuries. Adjust the depth and force of chest compressions accordingly to minimize further damage.

3. Abdominal Injuries

Patients with abdominal injuries may have internal bleeding or organ damage. While performing CPR, be cautious not to apply excessive pressure to the abdomen, as it can worsen the condition. Focus on maintaining adequate blood circulation and oxygenation without exacerbating the abdominal injuries.

4. Spinal Injuries

If there is a suspected or confirmed spinal injury, it is crucial to minimize movement and maintain spinal alignment during CPR. Use manual immobilization techniques or cervical collars to stabilize the head and neck. Coordinate with trained medical professionals to ensure the safest approach for the patient.

CPR for traumatic injuries requires a careful assessment of the situation, modified techniques, and special considerations. By understanding the unique challenges and adapting your approach, you can provide effective CPR and potentially save lives in these critical situations. Remember, every second counts and your quick response can make a significant difference in the outcome for the injured individual.

CPR in Drug Overdose and Poisoning

Drug overdose and poisoning are serious medical emergencies that require immediate attention and intervention. In these situations, performing cardiopulmonary resuscitation (CPR) can be a crucial step in saving a person's life. CPR in drug overdose and poisoning cases involves a combination of basic life support (BLS) techniques and specific considerations for the type of substance involved. In this section, we will explore the key aspects of CPR in drug overdose and poisoning scenarios.

Recognizing Drug Overdoses and Poisoning

The first step in providing CPR for drug overdoses and poisoning is recognizing the signs and symptoms of these conditions. Drug overdose can manifest in various ways, depending on the substance involved.

Common signs include unconsciousness, shallow or absent breathing, pinpoint pupils, seizures, and vomiting. Poisoning, on the other hand, can present with symptoms such as nausea, vomiting, abdominal pain, dizziness, confusion, and difficulty breathing.

Ensuring Safety and Activating EMS

Before initiating CPR, it is essential to ensure your own safety and the safety of others in the vicinity. If you suspect a drug overdose or poisoning, call emergency medical services (EMS) immediately. Provide them with accurate information about the situation, including the type of substance involved, if known. While waiting for EMS to arrive, it is crucial to stay with the person and monitor their condition closely.

Assessing the Person's Responsiveness and Breathing

Once you have ensured safety and activated EMS, assess the person's responsiveness and breathing. Tap the person gently and ask loudly if they are okay. If there is no response, check for normal breathing. Look, listen, and feel for any signs of breathing for no more than ten seconds. If the person is not breathing or is only gasping, it is necessary to start CPR immediately.

Performing Chest Compressions and Rescue Breaths

In drug overdose and poisoning cases, the primary focus of CPR is to maintain circulation and oxygenation. Begin by placing the heel of one hand on the center of the person's chest, slightly above the lower half of the breastbone.

Place your other hand on top of the first hand and interlock your fingers. Position yourself directly over the person's chest and, with straight arms, push hard and fast at a rate of about 100–120 compressions per minute. Allow the chest to fully recoil between compressions.

After performing 30 chest compressions, open the person's airway using the head-tilt and chin-lift techniques. Pinch the person's nose shut and create a seal over their mouth with your mouth. Give two rescue breaths, each lasting about one second, and watch for the chest to rise. If the breaths do not make the chest rise, reposition the person's head and try again.

Continue cycles of 30 compressions and two rescue breaths until EMS arrives or the person shows signs of life.

Special Considerations for Drug Overdose and Poisoning

When dealing with drug overdoses and poisoning, there are some additional considerations to keep in mind during CPR:

1. **Naloxone administration:** If the person has overdosed on opioids, such as heroin or prescription painkillers, naloxone can be a life-saving intervention. If you have access to naloxone and are trained to administer it, follow the specific instructions provided with the medication.

2. **Toxic substances:** Some substances can be harmful to the rescuer if they come into contact with the person's body fluids. Take precautions to avoid direct contact with the substance and use personal protective equipment if available.

3. **Poison control:** If the substance involved in the overdose or poisoning is known, contact a poison control center for guidance on specific treatment recommendations.

4. **Continuous monitoring:** While performing CPR, continue to monitor the person's vital signs and adjust your interventions accordingly. If the person regains consciousness or starts breathing spontaneously, stop CPR and place them in the recovery position.

CPR in drug overdose and poisoning situations requires prompt recognition, activation of EMS, and the application of BLS techniques. By maintaining circulation and oxygenation through chest compressions and rescue breaths, you can provide vital support until professional medical help arrives. Remember to consider any special circumstances related to the substance involved and take appropriate precautions to ensure your safety and the safety of others.

CPR in Hypothermia and Hyperthermia

Hypothermia and hyperthermia are two extreme temperature-related conditions that can have serious effects on the body. In both cases, the body's ability to regulate its temperature is compromised, leading to potentially life-threatening situations. As a CPR provider, it is crucial to understand how to perform CPR in these unique circumstances to increase the chances of saving a life.

Hypothermia

Hypothermia occurs when the body's core temperature drops below 95 degrees Fahrenheit (35 degrees Celsius). This can happen due to prolonged exposure to cold temperatures, immersion in cold water, or certain medical conditions. When a person is hypothermic, their body functions slow down, including their heart rate and breathing. In severe cases, they may even appear unconscious or have no signs of life.

Performing CPR on a hypothermic individual requires some modifications to the standard CPR techniques. Here's what you need to know:

1. **Assess the situation:** Ensure your safety and the safety of others before approaching the hypothermic person. If possible, move them to a warm and dry environment to prevent further heat loss.

2. **Activate emergency medical services (EMS):** Call for professional help immediately. Hypothermia is a medical emergency that requires specialized care.

3. **Check for signs of life:** Look for any signs of breathing or movement. If the person is unresponsive and not breathing normally, begin CPR.

4. **Modify chest compressions:** Due to the slowed heart rate in hypothermic individuals, it is recommended to perform chest compressions at a slower rate of about 80–100 compressions per minute. This allows for adequate blood flow without overwhelming the heart.

5. **Provide rescue breaths:** Deliver rescue breaths at a slower rate as well, aiming for one breath every 6–8 seconds. This slower pace helps to prevent the person from inhaling excessive cold air, which could further lower their body temperature.

6. **Monitor the person's temperature:** If possible, use a thermometer to monitor the person's core temperature.

This information can be vital for medical professionals when they arrive.

Remember, hypothermia is a serious condition, and the primary goal is to get the person to a medical facility as soon as possible. CPR is a temporary measure to maintain blood circulation and oxygenation until professional help arrives.

Hyperthermia

Hyperthermia, on the other hand, occurs when the body's core temperature rises above the normal range, typically exceeding 100.4 degrees Fahrenheit (38 degrees Celsius). This can happen due to prolonged exposure to high temperatures, strenuous physical activity in hot environments, or certain medical conditions. When a person is hyperthermic, their body's cooling mechanisms become overwhelmed, leading to heat exhaustion or heat stroke.

Performing CPR on a hyperthermic individual requires specific considerations to ensure their safety and increase the chances of successful resuscitation:

1. **Assess the situation:** Before approaching the hyperthermic person, ensure your own safety and remove them from the hot environment if possible. Move them to a shaded or air-conditioned area.

2. **Activate emergency medical services (EMS):** Call for professional help immediately. Hyperthermia can quickly escalate and become life-threatening.
3. **Check for signs of life:** Look for any signs of breathing or movement. If the person is unresponsive and not breathing normally, begin CPR.
4. **Modify chest compressions:** In hyperthermic individuals, the heart rate may be elevated. Adjust your chest compressions to a faster rate of about 100–120 compressions per minute to match the increased heart rate.
5. **Provide rescue breaths:** Deliver rescue breaths at a regular pace, aiming for one breath every 5–6 seconds. Be cautious not to provide excessive ventilation, as hyperthermic individuals may be more prone to lung injury.
6. **Cool the person down:** While waiting for professional help to arrive, take measures to cool the person down. Remove excess clothing, apply cool water or ice packs to their body, and use fans or air conditioning if available. However, avoid using ice baths or extreme cooling methods, as they can cause further complications.

Hyperthermia is a medical emergency that requires immediate attention. CPR should be performed until professional help arrives, but the primary focus should be on cooling the person down and preventing further heat-related complications.

By understanding the unique considerations and modifications required for CPR in hypothermia and hyperthermia cases, you can be better prepared to respond effectively in these challenging situations. Remember, always prioritize the safety of yourself and others, and activate emergency medical services as soon as possible.

CPR in the Elderly Population

As we age, our bodies undergo various changes, and our risk of experiencing a cardiac arrest increases. Cardiopulmonary resuscitation (CPR) plays a crucial role in saving lives, especially in the elderly population. In this section, we will explore the unique considerations and techniques for performing CPR on older adults.

Understanding the Aging Process

Before delving into CPR techniques for the elderly, it is essential to understand the physiological changes that occur as we age. Aging affects the cardiovascular system, making older adults more susceptible to cardiac events. The heart muscles may weaken, blood vessels may become less elastic, and the overall efficiency of the cardiovascular system may decline. These changes can increase the risk of cardiac arrest in the elderly.

Recognizing Cardiac Arrest in the Elderly

The signs of cardiac arrest in the elderly may differ from those in younger individuals. It is crucial to be aware of these differences to provide timely and effective CPR. Some common signs of cardiac arrest in the elderly include:

1. **Sudden loss of consciousness:** The person may collapse without warning.
2. **Absence of breathing or abnormal breathing:** The person may not be breathing at all or may have irregular, gasping breaths.
3. **Absence of pulse:** Check for a pulse at the carotid artery for at least 5 seconds. If no pulse is detected, it indicates cardiac arrest.

Performing CPR on the Elderly

When performing CPR on the elderly, it is important to consider their unique needs and limitations. Here are some key points to keep in mind:

1. **Gentle compressions:** Due to the potential fragility of the elderly population, it is crucial to apply gentle compressions during CPR. Aim for a compression depth of at least 2 inches, but be mindful of the individual's frailty and adjust accordingly.
2. **Positioning:** When initiating CPR, ensure that the person is lying on a firm surface. If possible, elevate the person's head slightly to open the airway. However,

be cautious not to hyperextend the neck, especially if there is a suspected neck injury.

3. **Compression rate:** The recommended compression rate for CPR in the elderly is the same as for adults, which is at least 100–120 compressions per minute. Maintain a steady rhythm and allow for full chest recoil between compressions.

4. **Rescue breaths:** Providing rescue breaths is an essential component of CPR. However, due to the risk of transmitting infections, it is recommended to perform compression-only CPR for bystanders who are not trained in CPR or are uncomfortable providing rescue breaths. If you are trained and comfortable, you can provide rescue breaths using a barrier device or a face mask.

5. **AED use:** Automated External Defibrillators (AEDs) are effective in restoring a normal heart rhythm during cardiac arrest. If an AED is available, follow the instructions provided and apply the pads to the person's chest as directed. Ensure that the AED is suitable for use with the elderly population.

6. **Considerations for frailty:** Frailty is common among the elderly and can affect their ability to withstand the physical demands of CPR. It is important to assess the person's overall condition and adjust the intensity of CPR accordingly. If the person is frail or has multiple

comorbidities, focus on providing high-quality chest compressions while minimizing the risk of injury.

7. **Communication and emotional support:** During a cardiac arrest event, it is crucial to communicate with the person and their loved ones. Offer reassurance and support, and keep them informed about the ongoing CPR efforts and the arrival of emergency medical services.

Remember, every second counts during a cardiac arrest, and initiating CPR promptly can significantly improve the chances of survival. By understanding the unique considerations and techniques for performing CPR on the elderly, you can play a vital role in saving lives.

Conclusion

Cardiac arrest can happen anytime and anywhere if the heart suddenly stops functioning. Without oxygenated blood flow, clinical death follows rapidly. The prompt provision of cardiopulmonary resuscitation is often the only chance for survival.

As outlined in this book, mastering CPR techniques empowers you to take decisive, lifesaving action when seconds count. By following the protocols for high-quality chest compressions, effective ventilation, proper AED usage, and pharmacological interventions, you maximize the chances of restarting the heart and preventing permanent organ damage.

Whether you use CPR skills as a medical professional or as a good Samaritan, routinely renewing your knowledge and skills is key. CPR guidelines continue to be updated based on the latest clinical research. Remaining current through retraining and practice with CPR manikins helps ingrain the techniques until they become second nature when emergencies strike.

By mastering CPR, you gain the ability to temporarily circulate oxygen until the heart can resume its critical pumping function. In the process, you bridge the gap between life and death for cardiac arrest victims. Though CPR is physically and emotionally demanding, few other skills provide a direct chance to save lives for both patients and loved ones. Your knowledge can ripple outward to equip entire communities to take action when it matters most.

During a cardiac crisis, the heartbeat of life fades rapidly without intervention. With the CPR techniques mastered here, you have the power to bring patients back from the brink and gift precious additional years to loved ones. Wield this knowledge with confidence to help fulfill CPR's ultimate promise: saving lives.

www.ingramcontent.com/pod-product-compliance
Lightning Source LLC
Chambersburg PA
CBHW070852260726
48661CB00004B/1375